The American Yoga Association's

Yoga for
Sports

The American Yoga Association's

Yoga for Sports

*The Secret to
Limitless Performance*

Alice Christensen

CB

CONTEMPORARY BOOKS

Library of Congress Cataloging-in-Publication Data

Christensen, Alice.
    The American Yoga Association's yoga for sports / Alice Christensen.
        p.   cm.
    Includes bibliographical references and index.
    ISBN 0-8092-2621-9
    1. Yoga, Hatha—Health aspects.   2. Athletes—Health and hygiene.
I. American Yoga Association.   II. Title.
RC1220.Y64C457   2000
613.7'046—dc21

                                            99-39627
                                              CIP

Reader's Note: The techniques and suggestions presented in this book are not intended to substitute for proper medical advice. Consult your physician before beginning any new exercise program or treating sports-related injuries. The author, the American Yoga Association, the producer, and the publisher assume no responsibility for injuries suffered while practicing these techniques. The American Yoga Association does not recommend this book for pregnant or nursing women or for children under 16 years of age. If you are elderly or have any chronic or recurring conditions such as high blood pressure, neck or back pain, arthritis, heart disease, etc., seek your physician's advice about which techniques you should avoid.

Interior photography by Evelyn England unless otherwise credited
Models' hair and makeup by Ashley Vann-Kingston
Cover design by Todd Petersen
Cover photograph by Herbert Ascherman, Jr.
Interior design by Hespenheide Design
Cover illustration by Dan Crovatin
Photograph, page 2, Alinari/Art Resource, NY
Photograph, page 7, The Metropolitan Museum of Art, Rogers Fund, 1914 (14.130.12)
Quote by Jack Nicklaus on page 9 excerpted with permission of Simon & Schuster, Inc., from *Golf My Way* by Jack Nicklaus with Ken Bowden. Copyright © 1974 by Jack Nicklaus.
Quote by Bill Bradley on page 17 from an interview with Michael Kelly. Originally published in *The New Yorker*.
Quote by Bill Russell on page 166 from *Second Wind* © 1979 (New York: Random House). Reprinted by permission of the author.
Quote by Bill Parcells on page 180 from *Finding a Way to Win* © 1995 (New York: Random House).

Published by Contemporary Books
A division of NTC/Contemporary Publishing Group, Inc.
4255 West Touhy Avenue, Lincolnwood (Chicago), Illinois 60712-1975 U.S.A.
Copyright © 2000 by The American Yoga Association
Printed in the United States of America
International Standard Book Number: 0-8092-2621-9

00 01 02 03 04 VL 19 18 17 16 15 14 13 12 11 10 9 8 7 6 5 4 3 2

This book is dedicated to my great teacher Rama. Even at the age of 72, he had the body of an athlete—perhaps a small prize-fighter. He possessed the extraordinary power of what is called *Laya*, the ability to maintain walking at a speed of approximately six miles per hour for endless periods of time. I had read of this Yogic feat in many old books in my Yoga studies over the years, but I had never seen it performed until I met Rama.

My students and I could never keep up with him. In fact, we used to line up on the front porch and set off in relays to see who could last the longest accompanying him in his morning "walk." He usually circled two or three blocks in our neighborhood in Cleveland Heights, enjoying the gardens and trees in the early dawn. One of us would be huffing and puffing along behind as he effortlessly sped along, laughing at us over his shoulder. One by one we would drop along the way and some other aspirant would take our place.

Rama stood out as a strange figure in the conservative section of Cleveland. In those days (the early 1970s), a golden-brown man flying along in a white muslin outfit that blew heartily in the wind was a sight that often brought an early dawn patrol car to his side to inquire if he needed a lift, whether "that person" (one of us) was chasing him or giving him trouble, and so on. He had many delightful conversations with the police explaining that he was from India where people walk most of the time and he was staying in practice for his return home. They would always ask about his life in India and tell him that at his age he ought to slow down a little and that they would be glad to drive him home.

Rama, who called everybody under 100 years of age "boy," would reply, "Oh, you boy! I need to enjoy my strength!" Then he would fly off on his legs, trailing a golden cloud of energy behind him.

CONTENTS

ACKNOWLEDGMENTS

I would like to express my deep gratitude to all the students, staff, and friends of the American Yoga Association for their help in the production of this book, particularly Pattie Cerar, Stephen R. Grant, and Patricia Rockwood. I would also like to thank our photographic models, all of whom enjoy sports of different kinds: Aireal Evans, personal trainer and in-line skater; Anne Ferrier, feng shui consultant and walker/weight trainer; Dale O'Hara, personal trainer and triathlete; Steve Honeyager, nursing student and martial arts practitioner; Artie Guerin, carpenter and tennis pro; and Lea Jackson, interior designer and swimmer.

Special thanks go to all the amateur and professional athletes who were kind enough to answer our many questions about their sport: Lemuel Andrews, high school basketball coach; Krista Benz, downhill skier; Peter Cerar, cyclist; Mike Colgrove, wrestler; Rick Dodson, gymnastics coach; Aireal Evans, in-line skater; LeeAnn Ferguson, ballroom dancer; Nelson Gonzalez, wrestler; Artie Guerin, tennis pro and former soccer player; Steve Honeyager, martial arts practitioner; Lea Jackson, former competitive swimmer; Alice Kennedy, basketball and volleyball player; Eve Kennedy, rugby and other team sports player; Bob Lape, race car driver; George Nodaros, archer; Dale O'Hara, triathlete; Barbara Porter, horseback rider; Rosemary Swain, dancer; Tommy Thompson, baseball catching coach; David Tipton, golfer; Elizabeth Walton, downhill skier; Tim Watnem, strength trainer; David Wilson, race car driver; and Marsha Wolak, tennis player. Besides being fascinating and insightful, their contributions add depth to the world of sport.

INTRODUCTION: A NEW APPROACH TO YOGA AND SPORT

Sports can send me on an emotional and physical roller coaster—from anger to sadness to pain to relaxation to euphoria. Sports, while physically taxing on the body, gives me an overall sense of my body being happy. My muscles are in tune and my body feels great. Then there are times when injuries occur and my body hurts or when the long practices tire me out. Depending on performance, my emotions can change from happiness to anxiety to sadness or anger. I have thrown things at lockers, I have jumped out of my chair in excitement, and I have sat in a locker room and cried.

—David Tipton

The language of sport is one of the few refuges of mythic consciousness in our culture's mainstream.

—Andrew Cooper,
Playing in the Zone

I have looked forward to writing a book on sports for everyone attempting the grand accomplishment of fusing the inner strength of the body with the outer physical form. The outer physical body is easily describable: it is the body that we can see and touch, which runs and speaks and breathes. The physical body has a consciousness all its own, which Yoga calls the physical ego. This is the aspect of consciousness that believes that the physical body is all there is. On the other hand, the inner-strength body, which I will be talking about throughout this book, is impossible to describe; the best way I can refer to it is as an emotional/spiritual/power body. These two distinct bodies exist in everyone, and it is possible to learn how to join them to make a whole that becomes greater than its parts. It is this union that becomes most usable to people in sport.

Throughout history—in sport, dance, drama, war, and play—we can see the astonishing phenomenon of the physical body reaching deep within itself to call on an unseen, extraordinary strength to accomplish heroic results. We look upon this type of phenomenon with awe, because it expresses a depth of strength and beauty that is not always seen in the physical body. It is indeed the mystical power strength that lies in the depths of the physical body, the individual's inner body of beauty and power, that the Greeks worshipped in the great games. Grecian society considered athletes as a physical representation of mythology, in which the divine energy of the soul was able to act through the athlete's body.

This inner beauty is powerfully portrayed in the statuary and art of the times. The miracle of great art astonishes us when the inner strength and beauty of the individual is shown radiating through the physical form. This is most often accomplished in sport.

> *I used to imagine myself seeing the pitch and hitting it the night before when I was going to bed. Seeing myself trying to be the hero, hitting the ball, winning the game. And then the actual next day somehow it all came into play and just happened the same way, which was kind of neat. I definitely did some of that.*
>
> —Tommy Thompson

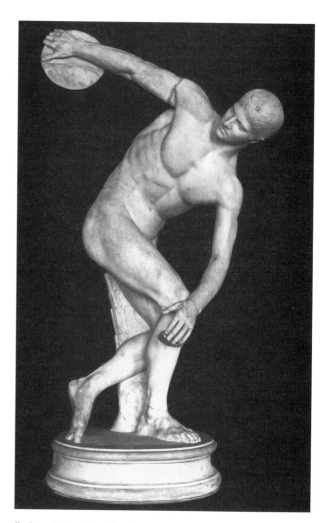

"Discobulus," a Greek statue created by Myron of Athens (5th c. B.C.E.)

As I mentioned previously, it is impossible to describe this unseen inner body with any precision. In this book I will call it the emotional/spiritual/power body. I use the term "emotional" because the inner body expresses itself through emotion. "Spiritual" refers to the inner intuitive voice of this body. "Power" refers to the extraordinary inner support that results when this body is joined with the outer physical body.

I find it amusing that the letters signifying the emotional/spiritual/power body are "ESP"—a flashback to the '50s and '60s when extrasensory perception was making headlines. However, this extra power given to a person by intuitive sources within is just what Yoga defines as realization of the inner self. It is indescribable, and it can express itself through the physical form. "Extrasensory perception" is a wonderful way to describe exactly what develops from the practices described in this book. "I've got more than I thought I had" and "I knew this was going to happen" are statements that illustrate the emergence of the intuitive awareness that personifies the inner power body—the extra force that, when called upon, comes forward to help you win the day. This information is not based on intellectuality; it is based on emotion.

Many athletes have described this type of experience when they speak of playing in the zone. For instance, Bill Russell, whose quote appears in Chapter 9, speaks of an unknown, indescribable power that sometimes takes over his play. It seems, from my many interviews with athletes, that almost everyone has experienced this feeling at one time or another. They all speak of it as an almost magical experience that is out of their conscious control.

Sometimes this inner body speaks to both players and spectators. The word *enthusiasm* comes from a Greek root meaning "possessed by a god"; in an enthusiastic game, both players and fans are carried away into a more primitive, ecstatic, and almost sacred state of being.

The physical body trains and prepares rigorously in every way to be able to perform, but there is a point when thought and body step aside and the inner spiritual/emotional power nature takes over. This inner body of the athlete then joins the outer physical body and is able to offer full strength to the performance. You cannot force this state. Artie Guerin, tennis pro and former soccer player, expressed it this way:

> To perform in sports, you have to have the fitness and you have to have the skill. But the key to performing in sports is not forcing yourself to do it, which is the best way to reach that state. If you say, "I've got to get in that zone, that focus state, I'm going to force myself to do it," then you're telling the physical body it's got to do it all and you're blocking out the spiritual side or voice.

Most of us never think about where the joy of running, throwing, or jumping originates. Classical Yoga would say that the origin is the emotional/spiritual/power body needing expression. An indescribable feeling comes to us when this expression takes form. The inner and outer bodies join, and the exhilaration of this feeling is so enchanting that athletes

are willing to face the pain of losing again and again in order to reach the state of feeling that allows them to achieve the impossible.

> *I had a friend/mentor who started doing triathlons at the age of 40. He lived with his wife and three children back in the woods in Nova Scotia. They self-taught their children and lived off the land as much as anyone that I knew of. I wanted to emulate him in every aspect, and when he spoke of the great mental and spiritual high that he got from completing triathlons, I knew I had to do one.*
>
> —Dale O'Hara, triathlete

The practice of breathing exercises is one way to help bring about this joining of the emotional/spiritual/power body with the outer physical body. I will talk more about how to practice breathing exercises later in the book.

The Importance of Ethics

The practice of ethics makes it easy to bring about the joining of the two bodies. The classical ideal of sport has always respected ethics as a way to approach this union. When ethical training is combined with physical training as a whole discipline, the athlete blooms with confidence.

Ethical training is generally ignored today. While it is true that ethical values help support society, I suggest that athletes practice ethics for individual purposes, such as greater self-confidence, freedom from fear, and improved present-moment awareness.

In Yoga, the practice of ethics includes 10 primary values. These are Nonviolence, Truthfulness, Nonstealing, periods of Celibacy, Nonhoarding, Purity, Contentment, Tolerance, Study, and Remembrance. At first glance, spending time in training on these values may not fit with your traditional view of sports training. In fact, sometimes ethical training has been considered as an inhibiting disturbance. In Yoga, however, ethics are not looked upon as restrictions on behavior, but as prescribed actions, all of which are performed for the sole purpose of increasing confidence and self-awareness. (For a more complete discussion of the ethics of Yoga, see my book *Yoga of the Heart*.) For instance, the ethic of Purity is very pertinent to athletes, because practicing this ethical behavior gives present-moment awareness. Present-moment awareness is essential to the heightened concentration and intuitive voice that is so necessary for most to achieve peak performance in any sport.

One of the ethical values stressed in Yoga that many people misinterpret is Tolerance. The Sanskrit word that is used in the original Yogic texts is *Tapas*, which is often translated as "asceticism" or "discipline," both of which usually have very harsh interpretations in the Western world. In the Yogic philosophy of Kashmir Shaivism, which is the tradition in which I have been trained, the word *Tapas* is translated as "Tolerance," which basically means, "You have reached your limit. Now take one more step." The great scholar and Shaivite master Lakshmanjoo, with whom I studied for nearly 20 years in Kashmir, constantly discussed these ethical principles with me in great detail. He pointed out that it is important to add, "How much can you stand happily?" There is no room for tortuous asceticism in Yoga. Discipline is taken on for growth and enjoyment, not for the sake of self-punishment. Athletes who remember to practice the ethic of Tolerance will never train in a self-punishing, self-destructive manner. Daily training becomes inviting.

Another significant benefit to athletes who add ethical training to their daily routine is increased self-confidence and self-esteem. Training in ethical values makes you feel good about yourself and is extremely helpful for athletic achievement. You are not afraid of loss or of making mistakes. The sense of inner pride and confidence in yourself protects you from crushing thought patterns such as "What if I lose?" or "What if I can't do it?" that can debilitate your efforts to succeed. Ethical practice supports you in all effort as you say to yourself, "I may have made a mistake, but I did the best I could under the circumstances and I am not ashamed of my effort." Someone who practices this achieves a great sense of inner pride and success that is not easily affected by outside criticism. Eve Kennedy, a young woman who plays many college team sports, said: "It drains you physically and emotionally when you lose because you spend so much energy trying to win. I do feel good, though, when I know that there is nothing more that I could have done in order to win. If I can walk off the court or field knowing that I personally put 100 percent of myself out there, then I feel that I have won."

One of the most important qualities for athletes is superb concentration. As I mentioned previously, concentration is one of the results of improved present-moment awareness, which is one of the effects of practicing ethics. Lakshmanjoo once told me: "The past is dead, the future is not yet born." He was referring to the space between thoughts, the source of concentration, the silence of the meditative experience (see Chapter 2). When you are not distracted by memories of the past or plans for the future, you can settle into a state of consciousness that is extremely restful and productive.

> The great Indian epic *The Mahabharata* tells of Arjuna, a prince whose real father was Indra, the god of thunder. Arjuna, like all his royal brothers, was born into the warrior class and spent his youth learning all the skills of warfare and strategy. He was an outstanding pupil and particularly excelled at archery. One day, the story goes, Arjuna and several of his cousins were practicing archery under the direction of their stern but beloved teacher, Drona. The boys took their positions, kneeling on the ground, bending their huge bows, and aiming for a bird in a tree several hundred feet distant. Drona asked each pupil what he saw. Some answered: "I see a wide field, trees bordering the field, and a bird in the tallest tree." Others answered that they saw only the tallest tree and the bird sitting in it. A few said that they saw only the bird. Finally Drona came to Arjuna, who said, "I see only the eye of the bird." Arjuna's ability to narrow his concentration to one point made him the hero of the day.

This is the only state in which intuition can come forward unhindered by the freight train of thoughts that constantly crowd our minds throughout the day. Intuition then speaks as the voice of the inner emotional/spiritual/power body. It puts you a step ahead of the game. One of the athletes we interviewed, Alice Kennedy, expressed it this way: "Playing any of my sports I have felt an almost euphoric stage. The best times are when I am playing and not thinking. When my body just knows what to do, which muscle to use, which way to turn, what shot to take. When I am not thinking, I am playing my best."

The Beauty of the Inner Body

I'm sure you know some people who have not been endowed with exceptional outer physical beauty but who actually shine with a different type of beauty from within. They radiate a power and warmth in their personality that completely negates the fact that they do not represent the common, marketable type of form and face seen in many advertisements. Instead, they present a completely different and unusual beauty in a natural way that makes the more commercial representation of beauty seem hollow and empty. In fact, marketing experts capitalize on this quality, searching for slight imperfections in the perfect look so that their resulting advertisement implies that there is more here than meets the eye. The attraction of the unseen beauty helps sell the product. Perfection cannot exist without imperfection, just as winning cannot exist without losing.

This is exactly the point in Yoga. The word *Yoga* means "to join or bridge." When a bridge forms between the physical body and the inner emotional/spiritual/power body, it creates a limitless power supply for the individual. The physical body is the vehicle that displays the inner body's expression, and it does so in a radiance and beauty that are unmistakable. An athlete who achieves this moment of joining shines with that power from within.

The idea of discovering your hidden quality is exactly what this book will be dealing with. Just as the extraordinary quality of beauty can be revealed in the example of commercial marketing above, the qualities of strength and excellence needed in sport can be brought forward in the individual in a dependable, usable form—always available, limitless, on call—to supply the beauty and excellence of movement in sport. Yoga looks upon this emotional/spiritual/power body as the total support of the physical body—indeed, the source of life itself.

A New Feeling of Wholeness

I have enjoyed sport all my life. I should explain, before going any further, that I consider sport to be the joy of using the body to achieve a desired goal. You may be surprised by this broad definition, but please read on. I think you will agree that mine is a very different outlook, one that you won't find among the vast number of books on sports that fill the shelves of libraries and bookstores throughout the world.

To reach any difficult goal, individuals need all the strength and cunning that is available to them. I offer a new way for you to train for sport that will give you a stronger and more complete feeling of wholeness to support whatever you want to do.

Everyone enjoys watching physical movement. It is pleasant to feel yourself involved with the movement you see taking place. You can project yourself into the feeling of movement and enjoy the involvement. It seems effortless because it is mentally based, and it allows perfect success in whatever you are observing, just as, in Thurber's famous story, Walter Mitty enjoyed elaborate fantasies of his involvement in various scenes of life.

It is easy to think of succeeding or winning when the effort is mentally based, but usually difficult to achieve with the physical body—and that's the fun of it! You pit yourself against yourself. You want to do it—but can you? The problem is that, in most cases, the emphasis in sport has been that you are pitting yourself against something or somebody else other than yourself. Yoga considers this outlook faulty because it moves your concentration away from yourself, thus causing an internal split of confidence and strength.

All practice in Yoga culminates when the physical body and the emotional/spiritual/power body join and become the complete support of the whole individual. You are trying to join forces with yourself. When this occurs, you can experience limitless ability: indefatigable, tireless, and unending. This is really what the joy of sport is all about: the realization that you can use your body to achieve a desired goal with beauty and excellence. This realization can be described as a remembrance of the divine ideal of the athlete; the return to your source.

These days, the world of sport does not encourage athletes to inquire within themselves. But the whole idea of returning to the divine ideal of sport rests on your ability to recognize total awareness centered in yourself. Your inner spiritual strength then combines with the physical to provide a limitless supply of extraordinary capabilities—so extraordinary, in fact, that they are constantly surprising. "Did I really do that?" is the astonishing statement made when this occurs. The challenge in sport is "How can I bring my full self together for the wholeness that is needed to show and enjoy the limitless potential that lies within me?"

The common avenue of approach to the inner body is usually a ruthless demand that it show itself and perform. After all my years of Yoga practice, I can tell you that this attitude may seem to show results, but these results are short-lived. The inner body that supports the physical and actually is the source of all your strength will retreat from such destructive handling. It stands aloof and has no need of egotistical show. I have learned over many years of practice that the best way to begin to know and appreciate the inner emotional/spiritual/power body is with affectionate, polite behavior. You may laugh about the prospect of pursuing part of yourself with polite behavior; however, the bridge between the two bodies—the inner and the outer—is fragile and delicate; it takes careful handling.

An affectionate, sensitive approach is needed, very similar to the gentle, supportive coaxing of a parent to a child as it matures. "I know you can walk. I know you can talk. You can do it. Now just try it again; you'll get the idea." All the basic qualities of the progenitor that encourage growth and mastery of the functioning physical body can be learned in childhood. But the child is not aware that the support of the physical body rests on the indescribable inner emotional/spiritual/power body. In fact, the child moves away from inherent knowledge of and natural bond with that support of the inner body with the growth of dependence on the physical body and the outside world. The child then must relearn awareness of and confidence in an inner body.

When the physical body learns to perform well, the scene can be reversed: the spiritual body becomes the parent, and the physical body becomes the child. The physical body looks for guidance and support from within, and the inner body supplies it willingly.

A necessary awareness of the two bodies will emerge; the premise of Yoga is that there can be no perfection in the physical body without this awareness. It is no longer "I have to do this"; instead it becomes "We can do this together." The physical body invites the emotional/spiritual/power body to show you new ways to function. The powerful inner body then is coaxed into displaying its glamour. The situation is no longer the fragile, lonely *I* of the physical but the strong support of the two halves of your body coming together in full strength. The soul of your body is then shown in all its beauty, strength, and poise.

This brings tremendous enjoyment. It displays itself in things that enhance the physical feeling of enjoyment, such as hitting that sweet spot on the ball, the feeling of a perfect dive, being able to hit the bull's-eye the first time—all things manipulable. The wonderful feeling of being able to do anything with perfection comes from the emergence of expression from the inner body. It brings with it a tremendous emotional confidence. The concentrated remembrance of this confident feeling can then accompany all motion—all action of the physical body. By doing this, you welcome and include the purity and strength of your inner body in your sport. You will have created an open road for its presence to show itself in all its power. No longer are you alone and vulnerable with your physical body. Something else is there: a powerful support body of excellence that offers strength and that, up to now, has only rarely been experienced.

This book will help you find companionship within yourself. Your whole self will emerge in a dependable, total strength performance. You will learn to create a constant bridge to your inner self just by remembering that it is there. When this takes place, wonderful self-growth and change occur, one of the most important being a change in your feelings about winning and losing.

> *No one loses in triathlons. Even if a first-timer records a DNF (did not finish), I feel the effort required to attempt such a physical challenge should be held in a high regard and viewed as a positive step.*
>
> —Dale O'Hara

Winning and Losing—A New Perspective

No one likes to lose. Everyone tries only to win. Losing, however, is important. Without losing, there would be no way to measure winning. It is the other half of a whole picture of sport.

Ancient Greek philosophy taught that the effort that goes into a game and the results, both winning and losing, are infused with what Carl Jung referred to as *mana*, a term he used to describe "an extraordinary effective power that emanates from a human being, object, action, or event, or from supernatural beings or spirits. Also health, prestige, power to work magic and to heal." This power, expressed in competition by early Greek athletes, was transformed into a store of blessings for all society, because both winning and losing represented the expression of the unseen inner body. All energetic effort in sport was considered heroic, because it was a representation of that body. That is the beauty of the athlete: the attempt to call on and express the unknown and do the impossible.

Winning and losing are a large part of sports. Tremendous pain is experienced in losing, and tremendous pain is connected with winning. Pain seems to be a part of the athletic experience. In fact, I have talked to many athletes who push their practices to a point of pain that seems unendurable, then try to pass that point into a type of euphoric consciousness in which the needs and discomfort of the physical can be ignored. These practices have devastating results on the body if practiced for long periods of time, and I think this is probably one of the main causes of burnout that plagues both professionals and amateurs. This, coupled with the fear of the emotional pain of losing felt by the disappointed fragile physical ego, sometimes keeps people from enjoying sports altogether. (The physical ego, as I explained previously, is an aspect of consciousness that believes the physical body is all there is.) This does not occur when the athlete is able to unite both bodies into a supportive force for the enjoyment of sport. Athletes can learn that the physical body is only the outer picture of their whole being. They learn by personal experience that they can contact the soul that lies deep within.

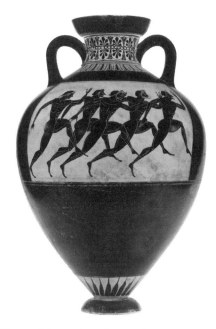

Black-figured Panathenaic amphora

The way you teach about losing is in the way you model it. When we lose a game, I try not to say anything to the guys at first. I let them just sit with their thoughts for a moment or so. And then I have to be careful what I say. Let them see that what I've been preaching I bring into the locker room after a loss. And then I'll say the same things to them. Well we did the best we could. We can improve on these areas. We'll come out tomorrow night and see how well we'll do. We'll work on these areas some more in practice. We learn. It's just a game. You've got to go on.

You know this year we had a guy who lost his brother, a young guy. He had been suffering with cancer but we didn't know that he was in bad shape because he was coming to all the games. So we thought maybe it was in remission. And then suddenly he's gone. His younger brother played on that team. This happened near the end of the season and gave us perspective. It made us a little bit more serious, at least for a couple of weeks there, just about life in general. Man, this is just a round piece of leather that goes through some nets.

—Lemuel Andrews,
high school basketball coach

I hope this book will show you how to develop a new personal attitude about yourself in sport that is based on solid building blocks of support that originate in yourself, melding two seemingly different systems—your inner and outer bodies—to join in a super-strong confidence of participation. I suggest you repeat this phrase daily: "I have the best chance of winning when I am in balance with my inner self. My inner emotional/spiritual/power body can supply all the power and strength I need." In other words, losing would not mean that you are a failure; instead it would be translated, "I was not able to put my physical ego out of the way so that my inner spiritual self could give me full power. I held myself back. My physical ego was in the way. I was out of balance. This can be fixed."

Lea Jackson, an athlete we interviewed who was a competitive swimmer as an adolescent, recalled her experience in a similar way: "Thinking back on it as an adult, I would say that whenever I lost it was because I got in the way. My ego probably got in the way of it. Because I remember having experiences where something else totally took over. And when that happened, generally I'd win."

This practice will reveal qualities you have at your disposal that your physical body has not used until now. Part of your preparation of your physical body for sport now invites the inclusion of your inner body in training. Using the two bodies together will supply the extraordinary ability to involve yourself totally in the enjoyment of any activity you choose.

In talking to people about their love of sports, I often ask them why they do it. They usually answer, "I don't really know; I just love the feeling of it." They do it, but they don't know why. This seems to be a clear statement that something unseen is operating. Making contact with the unseen part of yourself is the point of this book. The idea of excellence in sports is to join forces with yourself to present a strong, totally centered, whole being in full strength. I invite you to explore this idea with me in the following pages.

> *This is actually how I feel. This sport is not about winning or losing. It's nothing to do with that, and I can't even communicate what it is. This is me doing triathlons, but there are so many other people like me, and we don't know why we do it. I don't know why we subject ourselves to this.*
>
> —Dale O'Hara

1

YOGA FOR SPORT: THE BASICS

I never hit a shot . . . without having a very sharp, in-focus picture of it in my head. It's like a color movie. First I "see" the ball where I want it to finish, nice and white and sitting up high on the bright green grass. Then the scene quickly changes and I "see" the ball going there: its path, trajectory, and shape, even its behavior on landing. Then there is sort of a fade-out and the next scene shows me making the kind of swing that will turn the previous images into reality.

—JACK NICKLAUS,
Golf My Way

To me, golf is the ultimate challenge as a sport. Even though golf is a very competitive game when players play against one another, in the final analysis it is you playing in cooperation with and against yourself. Golf is very revealing as to your current mental outlook. If ever there was a sport where it can be said that you are your own best friend or your own worst enemy (sometimes both several different times during a round), golf is it. No two rounds of golf are alike, and each round offers something new to learn—about the game and about yourself.

—DAVID TIPTON

How Yoga Techniques Can Improve Sports Performance

As I stated in the Introduction, the definition of *sports* that I will be using throughout this book is any purposeful movement of the body, whether it be a walk around the block or a triathlon competition. Sports encourages enjoyable use of the body, and the total body performs best with a good maintenance routine.

Yoga exercises, called *asans*, are very efficient for this purpose. They consist of refined movements and positions that accomplish a wide variety of ends, including heart/lung conditioning, joint and muscle flexibility, back and large muscle-group strength, endocrine balance, and the health of both sympathetic and parasympathetic nervous systems. In other words, an asan routine affects every part of the body. A personal trainer we interviewed, Tim Watnem, mentioned something similar that happens in strength training: "You can look at the training as deliberately throwing your body into a fight-or-flight state. You're strengthening your sympathetic nervous system so it can go back to parasympathetic, the relaxation state, faster. Then when something happens, like somebody pulling in front of you in traffic, you recover a lot faster. So it saves your nervous system."

The most well-known use of Yoga exercise for athletics is as a warm-up tool, to improve flexibility by warming and lengthening the large muscle groups, stretching and increasing mobility in the spine, and stretching respiratory muscles to improve lung capacity. Balance and strength come easily when the whole body is exercised daily, and the Yoga asan routine can do it quickly and efficiently.

Asans support the day-to-day effort of athletic training by strengthening the body and central nervous system. At the same time, they promote changes in how we perceive ourselves and give a new awareness that makes training interesting. A well-rounded asan routine includes six broad types of asans: strengthening, stretching, balance, compression, inverted, and rest poses. Strengthening poses bolster our fortitude to persevere and to withstand. In balancing poses, the mind becomes highly concentrated, resolving into the silence of no thought. Stretching asans support the expansion of our awareness as we move beyond the limitations of our ordinary, habitual outlook. Compression poses produce intense inward focus, while inverted poses support the difference in perspective and outlook that comes as our awareness becomes more subtle. Finally, in rest poses, activity is brought to a single point of physical motionlessness, inner silence, and concentration.

> *Warm up and cool down are very important in all sports, but I think they are especially valuable in long-distance or endurance training. I always start slow and stretch to allow the muscle fibers to warm up before I get into the more intense part of the workout. To cool down I gradually allow my heart rate to slow down, and then I do another set of stretches. Keeping your muscles long and healthy through stretching and Yoga postures will prevent injury in any sport.*
>
> —Dale O'Hara

Asans are one of four major Yogic techniques at your disposal as an athlete. The second is breathing techniques, which are immensely helpful for improving stamina and concentration. Performing a brief set of breathing exercises just before competition can greatly focus your mind in a centered state where no energy is lost through distraction. This will also supply extra oxygen to the brain for performance.

The third technique is meditation, a gradual quieting of the mind until no thought remains. When this is done correctly, meditation results in a highly active inner awareness. Meditation brings on a subtle state of consciousness as the activity and restlessness of the mind subside into a profound and vast silence. When our mind steps aside from the physical ego during meditation, intuition—the voice of the emotional/spiritual/power body—is able to function clearly. A few minutes a day of meditation will also reduce accumulated stress and refresh and revitalize your entire being. Chapter 2, which teaches you specific breathing and meditation techniques, also discusses the benefits of these practices in more detail.

The fourth technique is visualization, or fantasy. Many athletes already use some sort of fantasy

ENERGY SOURCES FOR ATHLETES

Duration	Fuel	Activity	Yoga Helps
3-sec. burst	Cellular ATP	Power lift, high jump, shot put, golf swing, tennis serve	Balance musculature, stretch bulky muscles, improve cellular chemistry
8- to 10-sec. sustained burst	Cellular ATP and creatine phosphate	Sprints, fast breaks, football line play	
10- to 90-sec. sustained power	Muscle glycogen	200- 400-m dash, 50- 100-yd swim	
2 min. to exhaustion	Blood glucose and fatty acids from body stores	Runs beyond ½ mi. Continuous exertion	Increase breath volume and efficiency, store reserves, enhance recovery

All sport activity uses one of these four energy sources as the predominant fuel. Power molecules stored in the muscle cells mostly fuel short bursts of strength and speed, and as demands lengthen, the fuel source shifts to carbohydrate stores and then to stored fats and even body protein. This clearly shows the startlingly different demands various sports put on your body, even affecting cellular metabolism. Yogic routines are tailored to these different needs. Burst activities tend to create excessive bulk and strength in a few muscles leading to imbalance problems of pain and strain; Yogic routines balance and stretch, and improve cellular chemistry by improving circulation. For longer, endurance sports, burnout and breakdown are common adverse results as the body is repeatedly exhausted without proper attention to recovery. Yoga's restorative routines help. During performance, efficiency, especially that of breathing, is critical; Yogic techniques help to increase breath capacity, improving the body's ability to deliver oxygen to the working muscles.

exercise to prepare themselves for competition. In Yoga, the technique is used in conjunction with breathing exercises to improve self-confidence and to focus the mind. Visualization can give Yoga practice as well as your sports training a boost. My teacher Rama used to tell me that if I could not do asans physically, due to illness or travel, I should visualize myself doing them in my mind, and that the effect would be even stronger.

Visualization can be especially helpful in balancing unequal demands on the body. For instance, in a sport such as tennis, where one side of the body is used almost exclusively, fantasy can help to strengthen the nondominant side of the body, resulting in the athlete's ability to function with whole-body power. You will find specific fantasy suggestions in later chapters.

To prepare for each race, I would practice "bench driving." This term means simply sitting quietly alone somewhere and mentally "driving" the race course, corner by corner, lap after lap, mentally making every downshift of the gears, every brake application, every turn of the wheel, and every application of power to accelerate out of one corner and onto the next. You must be able to "drive" the entire race in your mind in order to actually drive the race on the track.

Winning is a goal of racing, and for some, it's the only goal. For me, however, running a good, clean race, at the limit of both my ability and that of the race car, was just as important to me as winning.

—Bob Lape, race car driver

What We Know About the Beginning of Yoga

Yoga is not a religion. Many people believe Yoga was derived from Hinduism, but this is not true. No one knows exactly when Yoga began, but evidence exists that it was practiced in India long before written history—long before the advent of the Hindu religion. Unlike religion, Yoga does not advocate rituals or creeds. It is based totally on individual experience. Yoga shows that very simple techniques, practiced in small increments, can bring realization of the fact that within our outer physical being is a universal spiritual nature that transcends the differences of social backgrounds, familial customs, and religious upbringing. The basic precept of Yoga is that this spiritual body support is the same in everyone and can be reached through simple daily practices.

The earliest practitioners handed down their knowledge orally from teacher to student, and this practice was carried on even after the advent of writing—in fact, it continues to this day. Only a few texts on Yogic philosophy remain from that early period, written in a sort of enigmatic code. More familiar to most of us are the many Yoga postures, or asans, which the early Yoga practitioners developed to keep their bodies in peak physical condition so they would have no distractions from meditative experience.

The Ethic of Nonviolence

Yoga has great respect for the physical body. It is recognized as the gateway for realization of the unseen inner being, which, in this book, I am calling the emotional/spiritual/power body. The physical body rests on the support strength of this inner body. As your practice becomes regular, you learn to listen and watch for its emergence. When you become familiar with its signals, you can gain great strength by combining the qualities of the inner body with your physical body's practice. Serious Yoga practitioners take great care not to harm their bodies. You may have seen pictures of so-called Yogis, emaciated with self-imposed starvation, lying on beds of nails or wrapped in thorn branches. These people are not really practicing Yoga; instead, they are practicing a form of religious asceticism

that denies the reality of the body and all other worldly things. Serious Yoga practitioners look upon these practices as self-violence. The body is your vehicle in this world. It is considered extremely precious and is used with care.

Nonviolence is the first and foremost of the ethical principles that Yoga students are encouraged to practice. I can guarantee that if you try even a little ethical practice, coupled with your daily routine, it will improve your performance greatly. The best way to begin is with yourself. Be good to yourself. Keep yourself healthy and strong by eating nutritiously, getting enough rest, and taking care not to injure yourself. When you train, be aware of your limits. Listen to your physical body tell you what it can and cannot do. Let your emotional/spiritual/power body tell you how to take care of your physical body and show you how to move toward perfection. You can attain a new awareness of your total self.

> *Fortunately, I have not been injured to the point where I must take extensive rest time. I try to keep my body in top condition by cross-training with weights and keeping my muscles long and healthy through stretching and Yoga. The most important advice I could give to anyone starting this sport is to listen to your body. When you are hungry, eat. When you are tired, rest. When you feel strong, go hard. When a muscle feels like it is going to explode, slow down or stop. You don't have to be a physical therapist to know how to stay injury-free. You have to establish a strong communication with your physical, mental, and spiritual sides.*
>
> —Dale O'Hara

If you are a serious athlete, you probably train hard, perhaps sometimes to the point of pain—or even beyond, into collapse and exhaustion. Violence to your physical body usually results in burnout or injury, which will not serve your desire for accomplishment in sport. In order to achieve excellence in your sport, the whole person must be involved and appreciated.

Practice Essentials

The only requirement for using Yogic techniques is the discipline of daily practice. This does not mean hours of practice; just a few minutes every day will yield tremendous results. The greatest benefit comes mainly from short daily practice. The results of Yoga are cumulative. Even 15 minutes of daily practice can be effective; if your time is extremely limited, any practice will show results. I find 30 minutes to be best as it gives time for meditation.

Yoga meditation will have the strongest effect when it is practiced after at least three asans. Many athletes prefer to split up their practice techniques, using Yoga asans for warming up before their workout and practicing breathing and meditation techniques at a later time; however, practicing asans and meditation together is best because of the effects of increasing glandular pressure during asan practice, which in turn affects meditation.

You should not practice Yogic routines immediately after eating a large meal or drinking caffeinated beverages. Wait an hour or so for best results. Yoga should never be practiced under the influence of alcohol or drugs. I have found that, as regular practice of Yogic routines is added to everyday discipline, the desire for the relief that drugs and alcohol bring fades away. The nondestructive source of relief is discovered within.

Asans should not be practiced by women during the heavy days of their menstrual cycle or during the first trimester of pregnancy. A limited routine of Yoga asans may be attempted after the first three months of pregnancy with your doctor's permission. (See the Resources section for books with more complete suggestions.) Meditation and simple breathing techniques are always appropriate, however, and, if practiced daily, will greatly improve the health and well-being of both mother and child.

You do not need any special clothing or equipment to practice Yoga. Wear any clothing that you like as long as it is loose or stretchy and warm enough for the season. Keep these clothes only for your Yoga practice. Practice asans barefoot so that you do not slip, but put on socks for meditation to keep your feet warm. As you meditate, your body temperature will drop slightly, so be sure to have a blanket or other covering available to avoid becoming chilled.

It is best to practice your Yoga routine on a mat, large towel, or blanket that you keep only for Yoga. Find a firm cushion or two that you can use for seated breathing exercises, and keep these separate also. This has a psychological effect: when you remember that these things are only for Yoga practice, it will help concentrate your efforts.

Overview of This Book

Because breathing and meditation training are important to all the sports discussed in this book, we have included detailed instructions for several techniques in Chapter 2. Chapter 3 teaches a core routine that can help every athlete by supplying a basic conditioning sequence of Yoga asans for strength, balance, and flexibility. Use this routine as your base, and add the particular techniques recommended in the chapter that covers your sport in more detail.

In the remainder of the chapters, we have loosely grouped sports according to the predominant movement or effort required. For instance, Chapter 4, "Target Sports," includes activities in which the goal is to hit a mark. As you prepare to throw a ball or shoot an arrow or take a jump, your focus is on the target. Many of the same sports fall into the category of activities that use one side of the body exclusively, such as tennis or bowling. This aspect of sports is discussed more fully in Chapter 5, which focuses on improving balance between the two sides of the body.

Chapter 6 includes any sport in which endurance is a factor, covering everything from cycling to basketball. Here you will find techniques to help improve stamina as well as performance. Chapter 7 covers sports that have a predominant artistic component, such as dance and figure skating. Although ballet, for instance, is sometimes considered more an art than a sport, a dancer must have a superbly conditioned body and the support of inner strength in order to succeed, and many of the techniques of Yoga can help achieve this goal.

Sports that require strength and balance are included in Chapter 8. Team sports are individually covered in chapters 4 through 8 as appropriate, but we offer a special discussion in Chapter 9 about how Yoga can help empower the team by improving intuition and communication. Finally, in Chapter 10, we

CARBOHYDRATES

Athletes have increased energy requirements compared to the general population. Carbohydrates are the preferred fuel of all sports activity. If you make only one change to your sports diet, it probably should be to increase carbohydrates to 60 percent of total calories. More than 95 percent of athletes, however, do not eat close to the U.S. dietary goal for carbohydrates for the general public, much less the higher dietary goal for athletes. Women athletes are notorious for avoiding carbohydrates because of a mistaken belief that they are fattening, and men tend to avoid them in favor of high-fat junk foods. High-carbohydrate foods are the best choice to provide the extra calories required to support training and competition activities, and this increased carbohydrate intake automatically increases the consumption of essential vitamins and minerals. (For best carbohydrate sources, see sidebar, page 18.)

offer some words to coaches about how they can use Yoga techniques both to improve their own health, well-being, and understanding and to encourage and inspire the athletes in their care.

Nutrition and Sports

No book on sports performance would be complete without information on nutrition. Both professional and amateur athletes need the support of a balanced, healthy diet. Eating right is an important way to practice nonviolence toward yourself. Nutritional information is sprinkled throughout this book. You will find suggestions for how to get enough carbohydrates, suggestions about the best snack foods, the truth about "sports drinks," food supplements, and much more. We have not included specific menus and dietary recommendations in this book; however, there are a number of excellent books on the subject, and we have listed several in the Resources section at the end of this book.

If You Want to Learn More About Yoga . . .

In this book we have room only for a brief introduction to Yoga. If you decide you'd like to find out more, see the Resources section for a complete list of other books and tapes by the American Yoga Association, as well as information on how to contact us. Please feel free to write to me if you have any questions or comments about what you are doing.

2

BREATHING AND MEDITATION: THE FOUNDATION OF PERFORMANCE

Mental and physical conditioning are as important to a race car driver as to a tennis player, golfer, or team-sport player. Many of the races in which I participated were "endurance" races of 6-, 12-, even 24-hour durations. Endurance racing requires codrivers, who take turns behind the wheel at two-hour intervals, night and day, around the clock. Driving a typical road race course at night requires unbelievable focus.

Since I have retired from active racing, I can only speak of such things as goals and progress in the past tense. I don't consider myself a good athlete. At age 45, I chose a

sport where I had to compete with teenagers. I can't think of one other sport (football, basketball?) where someone that age could compete with youngsters. In racing, you do. I was so focused on learning the skills of being a race driver, I was able to overcome my natural athletic limitations. Although it took a couple of years, I honed my driving skills and became a consistent driver, finishing first, second, or third in nearly every race. My determination to excel at something seemed to keep me focused on my objectives.

—BOB LAPE

There are several ways in which the Yogic techniques of breathing and meditation can be helpful to all athletes.

Benefits of Breathing and Meditation

Improve Focus and Concentration

Athletes realize the importance of achieving and maintaining a high level of concentration in order to perform at their best. Yogic breathing and meditation techniques can give you an easy way to reach intense concentration.

When you practice breathing techniques correctly, all your attention is focused on the breath, specifically on the sound of the breath as you slowly breathe in and out. Meditation training begins with a step-by-step guided relaxation process in which you focus on each part of your body individually to relax it. When the two techniques—breathing and meditation—are practiced together, intense concentration takes place automatically. This concentrated state is then used to shift your mental focus to a completely silent state in meditation. It can be described as a time of no thought. Several athletes who practice Yoga have talked about the similarity of this silent state to what they experience at the peak of their effort in sport.

Help Manage Stress Before Competition and Throughout Daily Life

No one is completely free from precompetition jitters. A little anxiety before performance often can help you by providing a slight adrenaline push to your body and by stimulating you to focus in order to do your best. Too much anxiety, however, drains your body of strength and makes it harder to concentrate. Learning to use Yogic breathing techniques to reduce your anxiety before competition can make the difference between a great performance and a mediocre one.

Breathing and relaxation training can help you manage stress in other areas of life as well. Try the Complete Breath technique (page 20) when facing a difficult situation at work, during uncomfortable medical procedures, when worried about finances or

> *I would do deep breathing exercises that my mom showed me to calm myself down before a game or to catch my breath during a game. I would also use breathing as part of my serving, batting, and foul shot routine.*
> —Alice Kennedy

relationships, or when late for an appointment. If you have trouble getting to sleep or staying asleep, go through your complete relaxation and meditation procedure lying in bed. You will fall asleep easily without the need for medication.

Build Stamina, Increase Vital Capacity, and Stretch Respiratory Muscles

Sports require a greater breath capacity than most people develop naturally. Regular practice of breathing exercises will help to increase your lung capacity by stretching all the respiratory muscles and teaching you to breathe deeply, even when you are not exercising. Oxygen levels in the brain are then maintained for highest efficiency.

Return to a Resting State More Quickly

When you are very active, it is important to be able to rest as quickly and completely as you can. Regular practice of the relaxation and meditation technique trains your body and mind to relax at will, allowing you to rest and recharge more efficiently and more quickly.

Increase Self-Confidence

Nothing gives a competitive edge like self-confidence. When you know that you are able to perform at your best, you don't need anyone else to tell you so. Self-confidence is increased when you welcome the participation of your emotional/spiritual/power body; self-confidence goes out the window when you think everything depends on the physical body alone. I have included the "I Love You" meditation technique in this chapter because it is one of the best ways I have found to instill and maintain confidence in yourself.

After that first year with the Knicks, with the way the public, the audience, treated me, I always had a great deal of ambivalence, and therefore I never gave myself to the public. And as a result, you know, I came to feel that it was my performance on the court and the integrity of what we were doing there in and of itself that mattered, and that the millions watching were incidental to what the craft was—and that realization was a liberation.

—Bill Bradley

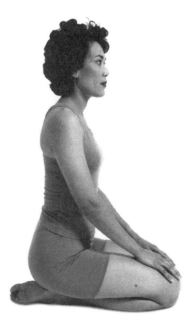

Figure 2.2

Breathing Techniques

We begin with a few techniques you can do sitting in a chair or kneeling on the floor to warm up the respiratory muscles, which include the muscles between your ribs, your abdominal and lower back muscles, and the muscles that criss-cross your torso. Practice these exercises before your warm-up routine, before performing the Complete Breath, and at other times of the day for a refreshing lift.

Breathing exercises can be done sitting on the edge of a straight chair with feet flat on the floor (Figure 2.1) or sitting on the floor, either cross-legged (Figure 2.2) or sitting on folded legs (Figure 2.3). Note that the model in the cross-legged photo is sitting on a cushion. A small, firm cushion will keep your back straight and less fatigued, especially if your knees and hips are stiff.

Always breathe through your nose, both inhaling and exhaling. This allows you to breathe more slowly and deliberately and, more importantly, it gives you an easy point of focus: the sound of the breath. If you concentrate on the sound of the breath while you do these exercises, you will soon find that

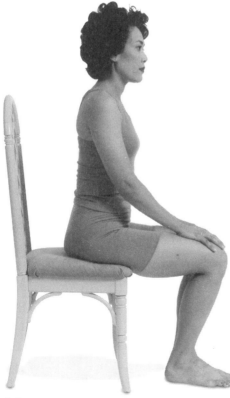

Figure 2.1

Figure 2.3

you are not able to think about other things, which makes the technique much more effective and contributes greatly to the stress-coping effect. Naturally, if your attention is completely focused on one thing, namely the sound of the breath, you won't be able to simultaneously think about finances, family problems, competition anxiety, or any other distraction. It gives your mind a rest.

If you close your throat very slightly, you will notice a distinctive sound made by your breath; it is somewhat like making the sound of the letter h but with your mouth closed. Concentrate on this sound as you breathe, and breathe as slowly as you can without gasping for air.

It is best to breathe through both nostrils. If you find that one nostril is closed, put pressure in the opposite armpit with your fist (for example, if your right nostril is closed, press into the left armpit with your right fist). After you have held your fist firmly in your armpit for a minute or two, the blocked nostril will open.

Frog Pose

Sit straight, either in a chair or on the floor in one of the positions described above. Place your hands on your knees. Breathe in deeply through your nose as you arch your back and look up, leaning forward slightly (Figure 2.4). Hold for a moment. Breathe out through your nose as you bend the opposite way,

> ### BEST FOOD SOURCE: CARBOHYDRATES
>
> Eat fruits, vegetables, and grains! This is the best way to fuel your body for exercise. Boosting carbohydrates to 60 percent of total calories increases stamina and decreases recovery time after exhaustion. Apples, oranges, bananas, and raisins are some excellent fruit choices, and starchy vegetables such as corn, winter squash, potatoes, beans, peas, lentils, and carrots are loaded. Grain foods such as bread, crackers, pancakes, and breakfast cereals are great choices too, especially if they are made from whole grain.

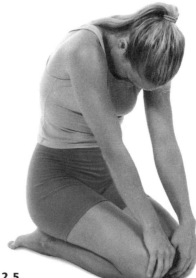

Figure 2.5

rounding your back and tucking your chin into your chest (Figure 2.5). Hold for a moment. Repeat twice more.

Side Stretch

Sit straight in a chair or cross-legged on the floor. Let your arms relax at your sides. Take a deep breath in and bend toward your right side, stretching your right arm down toward the floor and bending your left arm

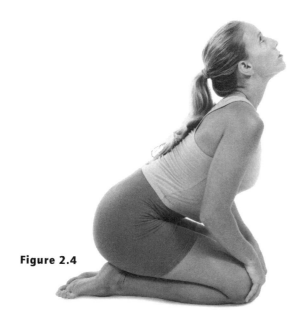

Figure 2.4

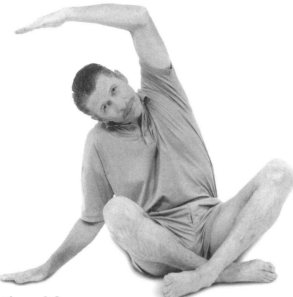

Figure 2.6

up and over your head (Figure 2.6). Hold for a moment. Breathe out and return to your starting position. Repeat three times on each side, alternating.

Arm Swing

Sit straight in your chair or on the floor. Stretch your arms straight ahead, level with your shoulders, and breathe out (Figure 2.7). Start to breathe in deeply

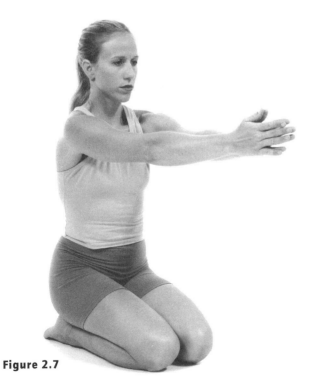

Figure 2.7

and push your chest and stomach forward as you open your arms wide to the sides and back as far as you can behind you without straining (Figure 2.8). Breathe out as you slouch forward again, and bring your arms together in front of you. Repeat three to five times, slowly.

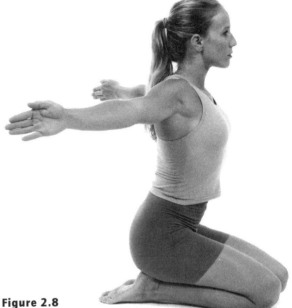

Figure 2.8

The next two breathing techniques help you breathe more deeply and completely by teaching you to use your diaphragm fully.

Belly Breath

This exercise, which you can do in almost any position, will help you become more conscious of the function of your diaphragm. The Belly Breath is especially helpful if you have trouble going to sleep. It can also help calm excess anxiety before performance or in any stressful situation.

To make the exercise easier to learn the first time, sit on the edge of a chair with your feet flat on the floor. When you have learned the exercise, you can practice it seated on the floor in whatever comfortable position you like. You can also practice this breathing exercise almost anywhere: lying in bed, in the car while waiting for a light to change (please do not practice while actively driving!), in a waiting room at the bank or doctor's office, or standing in line.

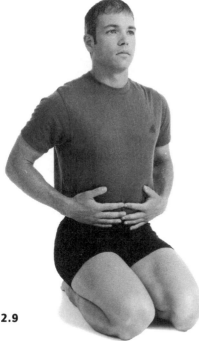

Figure 2.9

Complete Breath

In the Complete Breath, the movement of the Belly Breath is extended up into your ribs, where you expand the muscles between your ribs, and finally your chest, where you push air into the topmost sections of your lungs.

Learn the exercise seated on the edge of a chair with feet flat. You may switch to a seated position on the floor later, but be sure to sit on one or two firm cushions to raise your hips and prevent tension or slouching in your lower back. Always breathe through your nose, and concentrate on the sound of the breath as described on page 18.

Place your hands on your belly and breathe out, trying not to slouch forward. Tighten your belly muscles to get as much air out as possible. Now begin to breathe in from the bottom up, letting your belly muscles relax so the air appears to fill your belly. What you are actually feeling as your belly relaxes is your diaphragm expanding fully, allowing oxygen into the entire lower section of your lungs.

Continue to breathe in and feel the air filling the center part of your torso. Imagine the muscles between your ribs stretching so that your ribs expand in all directions, not just forward. Breathe in a little more and feel the air filling the very top sections of your lungs (Figure 2.10). Do not hold your breath,

Place both hands on your abdomen just below your navel (Figure 2.9). This is the part of your body that should move as you breathe in and out—not your chest. Remember always to breathe through your nose. Start by breathing out completely. As you breathe out, tighten your belly muscles and pull in with your hands to reinforce the movement. You should notice that the muscles along the sides and back of your torso will also contract. Try to get as much air out as possible without straining or curving your back forward; your back and shoulders should remain straight throughout the exercise. Start to breathe in and release the pressure on your belly; notice that your belly begins to fill of its own accord. Breathe in as much as possible, then start to breathe out again as before. Repeat the cycle five to ten times.

> *When I train I almost go into a meditation with my breath work. I go into a state that is a kind of "high." It's like getting a lot of oxygen and releasing endorphins, kind of a runner's high. Combined with the breath work and the pushing of the muscle, the flow of blood, I get really high and even more focused on what I'm doing. That's what I would call peak performance.*
>
> —Tim Watnem

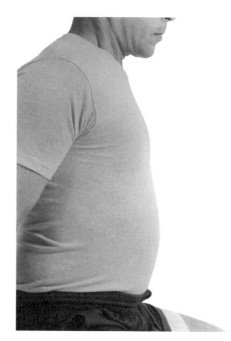

Figure 2.10

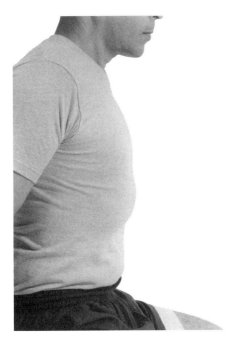

Figure 2.11

Relaxation and Meditation

Complete Relaxation Procedure

This simple procedure teaches you how to relax your entire body, step by step. It is really important to learn this technique before going into meditation, because you can't truly concentrate on what's happening in your mind if your body is tense or uncomfortable. Yoga asans were developed to keep the body healthy and strong so that aches, pains, and discomfort would not intrude on meditation. A cassette tape of this procedure is available from the American Yoga Association; see Resources for details.

To get the most from meditation practice, follow these suggestions:

1. **Find a comfortable position.** We recommend that you begin relaxation and meditation practice lying down because you won't have to worry about maintaining an erect posture or about your knees, hips, and back becoming stiff and distracting you (Figure 2.12). The position is called the Corpse Pose. You can also meditate in a seated

but gently start to breathe out, slowly, from the top down. First relax your chest, then let your ribs contract, and finally tighten your belly and push the last of the air out (Figure 2.11). Do not hold your breath at the bottom of the cycle either. Repeat the Complete Breath three to ten times.

Depending on your current breath capacity, the complete cycle of the Complete Breath (one inhalation, one exhalation) may take 10 to 30 seconds. It is important to breathe in and out for approximately the same length of time. Most of us naturally breathe out longer than we breathe in. In the Complete Breath you are counteracting that tendency and breathing more evenly.

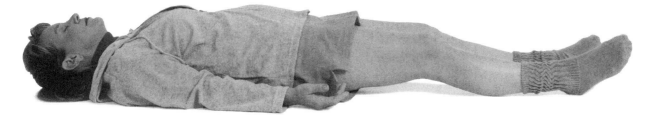

Figure 2.12

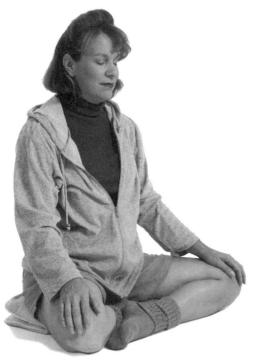

Figure 2.13

position, supported by a firm cushion, if you are very comfortable. The test is whether your knees rest on the floor when you are sitting cross-legged (Figure 2.13).

2. **Stay warm.** Wear socks and wrap yourself with a sweater or shawl. Even if you feel warm from exercising, the stillness of relaxation and meditation will result in a slight drop in body temperature, and it is important to avoid becoming chilled.

3. **Protect yourself from disturbance.** Ask your family not to interrupt you during this time, and make sure pets are in another area. Turn off your telephone. Keep your practice space quiet; do not play music during any part of Yoga practice.

This complete relaxation procedure will take between 5 and 15 minutes. If there are times when you wish to practice but cannot spare that amount of time, use the Quick Relaxation procedure described on page 24.

Read over the following directions and then close your eyes and begin relaxing. You will be focusing your attention quietly on each part of your body, visualizing each part in turn without moving any part of your body except your breath. Simply tell yourself to relax each body part in your mind.

Start with your face. Gently and calmly bring all of your attention to your forehead. Feel all of the muscles in your forehead. Let them relax so they feel loose.

Become aware of your eyes. Are they tense and jumpy? The eyes are usually the most difficult body part to relax, so just let them loosen and float in the sockets. Let all tension and movement in the eyes stop. Move on to your lips, teeth, and all the muscles of the jaw, mouth, and throat. Let your tongue relax in your mouth, and say to yourself, "I don't have to speak for a few minutes." Feel all the skin on your face become loose. Let your scalp relax and imagine your ears drooping toward the floor. Your eyes may continue to jump around a little, but after regular practice you will be able to relax them more and more.

Now relax your shoulders, arms, and hands. Imagine that your arms are hollow. Let all the muscles of the shoulders settle loosely on the floor. Move down into your elbow joints and imagine you can see and feel the bones. Relax and loosen them. Do the same with your forearms, wrists, and right into your hands and fingers, making them hollow and loose. Relax your fingers completely as though they were empty gloves lying on the floor.

Silently move your attention, like a tiny, warm relaxing beam of light, into your chest and, for a few moments, just observe the air moving in and out of your lungs. Feel your heart beating softly and rhythmically. Notice your belly rising and falling as you breathe. Do not try to speed up or slow down your breathing. Instead, just picture your lungs. Then take in a gentle breath of air, and, just as though you are sighing, let the breath out and relax your lungs. Take in another deep, gentle breath, sigh it out, and feel your heart relaxing also. Then let go of your breathing altogether, and relax all tension or effort in your breathing. Observe your belly and try to relax the squeezing effort as you breathe out. Each time you exhale, make your breath as relaxed as possible so that you are exerting almost no effort to breathe.

Now move your attention down into your legs, picturing them hollow, just as you did with your arms. Loosen and relax your thighs, hip sockets, and groin. Relax your knee joints until you feel as though your lower legs are also hollow and empty, all the way into your toes. Imagine that your feet are empty—nothing inside, not even any bones. Feel your toenails relax and loosen.

Move up inside your empty feet, legs, and thighs, and bring your attention to the base of your spine. As you move upward through your waist area, relax any sign of tension so that your entire spine feels rubbery and loose. Feel your spine and all of its joints all the way up to the base of your skull. Spend a little extra time at the back of your neck. This common tension site needs extra attention. Imagine you can look right down inside your spinal column as though your spine were a rope dangling down into a dark well. Relax your spine until it feels as loose as that rope.

Next, concentrate on moving inside your head. Bring your attention back to your face to check whether or not your face is tense. Relax your eyes even more now, and let them float almost as though you can't feel them move at all.

Recheck the three main tension areas.

1. **Is your breathing relaxed?**

2. **Are your eyes and facial muscles relaxed?**

3. **Is the back of your neck relaxed?**

Your body will eventually feel as if it were just an empty shell with no tension anywhere. The only movement will be your heart and your breathing, but they also will be very relaxed. Now relax the entire inside of your head. Feel your brain quietly settling inside your head with no effort or strain—just quiet and still.

Here is a summary of the relaxation steps:

1. Relax your face and eyes.
2. Relax and empty your arms and hands.
3. Relax your lungs and heart.
4. Relax your belly and breathing.
5. Relax and empty your legs and feet, especially your thighs and knees.
6. Relax and loosen your back, shoulders, and neck.
7. Relax the inside of your head.
8. Recheck the three major tension areas: your face and eyes, your breathing, and the back of your neck.

On the days of long, slow training where I know I will be out there for a few hours, I practice slowing my breathing down and trying to get into a meditative state.

—Dale O'Hara

Meditation

Now you are ready to meditate. Meditation is not concentrating on your breath, or a sound, or anything else; it is simply no thought. For 10 to 30 minutes, try not to think about anything. Most people find this difficult at first, but if you try every day, it will become easier and more rewarding. The constant barrage of anxieties, plans, self-recriminations, and other thoughts that flow through our minds daily are a prime source of stress. Learning to release those thoughts will greatly improve your stress resistance and increase the energy and strength you have for your athletic activities.

Start your meditation period by thinking of the sound *Om* (pronounced "ohm"). This word is a sound formula that has a specific effect on the mind when it is repeated or heard. *Om* is the oldest and most basic sound in classical Yoga. It has been said that if you could hear the subtle humming sound of the collective atomic structure of your own body and mind, that sound would most resemble the sound *Om*.

The *Om* sound of classical Yoga has been adopted and used in a religious way by nearly every religion of the Eastern world. However, in classical Yoga, the sound *Om* is used to center and focus the mind, and is not meant to indicate any particular religious concept or deity. Its purpose is to empty the mind except for the sound itself, leading finally to complete silence.

When you practice meditation, you will probably find that your experience of silence will be deeper and more refreshing if you repeat the sound *Om* to yourself several times at the beginning of your meditation session. Then simply stop talking to yourself in your mind. Try to stop all inner conversation. Don't force it; you will probably be quiet for a few seconds, then a thought will come into your mind. It may be several more seconds before you realize that you are thinking again. When you do notice that you are thinking, just let the thought trail away in your mind and go back to the experience of silence. This will happen several times during your meditation period and it is perfectly normal; meditation is a process, not a forced goal to add more stress to your life!

When you begin to understand this, you will never find yourself saying "I had (or didn't have) a good meditation today." It is a process without a standard for comparative judgment. Treat your daily meditation session like a game; see how long you can be still before a thought interrupts you. Some days you will be able to be still for a long time; other days it will be difficult to stop talking to yourself or even stop thinking even for a second. Just keep trying every day and focus on the refreshing, quiet feeling that stays with you after your meditation session.

Eventually you will notice that this feeling will accompany you throughout your day. All you have to do is remember the feeling and it will be there. Many students tell me that their daily meditation period is as refreshing as taking a short nap. It is a tremendous help to concentration.

Don't worry if you fall asleep during meditation at first. This is natural, because your body is receiving all the normal signals of sleep: eyes closed, body relaxed, and so forth. Just keep meditating and eventually your body will learn to rest deeply while your mind remains alert and focused on silence.

Decide before you start meditation how long you are going to remain quiet. For best results, try to meditate for at least 10 minutes at first. Later, when the process becomes more comfortable, you can extend your meditation period to 20 or 30 minutes, or even longer if you wish.

After Meditation

The way you come out of meditation is as important as how you relax into it. If you get up too quickly, or disturb yourself too abruptly, you may feel irritable or upset. Before you start to move around, open your eyes and lie still for a few minutes longer thinking about the sensations, feelings, and thoughts you experienced during your meditation period. Then increase your breathing a little, and that will start to reactivate the rest of your body and consciousness. At first, when you go to move your hands and arms, they may feel a bit wooden since they've become so

> *I visualize on the fibers, the muscles. I visualize the fibers actually sliding together and extending apart; contracting and extending. Sometimes I'll visualize just my breath. The intake of oxygen is like a transport of oxygen to that muscle. So when I'm strength training, I'm concentrating on bringing oxygen to that muscle in order for that muscle to grow. I'm picturing the blood and oxygen flowing to the muscle.*
>
> —Tim Watnem

utterly relaxed. Make fists of your hands; then release them. Keeping your legs straight on the floor, flex your feet back toward your chin and then point them away. Do this a few times. Stretch your arms and legs like a cat does when it awakens from a nap. As you move toward your normal activities, you will feel refreshed, alert, and recharged with new energy and a clear mind.

Quick Relaxation

Sometimes you may want to meditate but have only a short amount of time in which to prepare. The following quick relaxation can be used at these times to help you enter the quiet feeling of meditation more quickly.

Start by lying on your back on your mat, with legs a few inches apart and arms at your sides, palms facing up. All at once, tighten all the muscles of your body and lift up so you are balancing on your buttocks. Then release and let your body fall back to the floor. Shake each limb in turn: left arm, right arm, left leg, right leg. Roll your head gently from side to side. Shake your entire body gently and feel the sensation of melting into the floor. Take a deep, slow breath in, then release it all at once and relax your breath. With your eyes closed, go on to the meditation instructions.

"I Love You" Meditation Technique

One of the most important qualities for an athlete is self-confidence. This technique is the best way I have found to build a solid foundation of self-confidence from the inside out. This technique, practiced regularly, will help to reinforce feelings of self-confidence, raise self-esteem, and remove fear. This technique should be done as a complement to—rather than as a substitute for—your daily meditation session as described above.

Start with the Laughing Bicycle (Figure 2.14): Lying on your back, pump your legs as though you were riding a bicycle. Pump your arms as well, and laugh out loud for several seconds. Enjoy feeling foolish. Then relax and settle into the Corpse Pose. This exercise helps to release tension and stimulates the brain chemicals that cause feelings of well-being. A cassette tape of this technique is available from the American Yoga Association; see Resources.

Prepare for the technique just as if you were about to meditate: Lie on your back comfortably, without a pillow under your head, on your bed or the floor, or in a chair in which your back remains straight. Keep yourself warm with a blanket or shawl. Make sure your pets are in another room, and turn off your telephone. Press your back slightly toward the floor, then release and relax. Pull your chin down a little toward your chest without straining, to stretch the cords in the back of the neck that will allow more movement of the feeling that is going to affect your brain. If your lower back is tense, place one or two pillows under your knees.

Bring your attention to your forehead. Breathe in, saying "I love you" to yourself. Do the same as you breathe out. Repeat several times: breathe in "I love you" and breathe out "I love you." Breathe in

and hold for a moment. Imagine the feeling "I love you" spreading throughout your brain in a beautiful, warm, wet, perfumed essence. Breathe out "I love you."

Relax completely. Let your breath relax. Hold that feeling. Then, for a few more minutes, continue saying "I love you" each time you breathe in and out.

As you breathe in and hold your breath for a moment, think to yourself, "Whom do I love?" Breathe out and say "I love you." Breathe in and hold again; think: "Who loves me?" Now think to yourself: "My breath loves me." Breathe out. "My breath loves me." The breath is inside you. It loves you. Breathe in and think "I'm holding my breath—it loves me." Breathe out and think "I have released my breath—It still loves me." Take a deep breath, always through your nose. Breathe in: "My breath loves me." Breathe out: "My breath is gone now, but it still loves me."

Now relax completely. Visualize the inside of your head and your body. Think of the breath commingled with love. Oxygen is flowing through your arteries and heart and every part of you because you can't live without your breath. Visualize this loving breath inside your body. Are there any blocks keeping it from moving where it wants to go? Visualize this feeling of love and breath removing any kind of constriction, moving easily and sweetly throughout your body.

Bring the feeling to your forehead. Think "I love you—my breath is in my forehead." Relax your forehead. Now think of this feeling of love spreading to your eyes—you can almost see it! Relax your eyes and let the breath of love simply swim out into the rest of your face. Feel this breath of love in your nose, because it breathes for you. Every time you breathe in, breathe "I love you." Every time you breathe out, breathe "I love you." Let the breath of love flow freely so that your face melts with love. Let your mouth and throat relax, thinking "I love you" as you breathe.

Let your neck relax now so you have no constriction that will stop the breath from moving. Love comes in with your breath—relax. Love goes out with your breath—relax. Drop your collarbone toward the floor and say "I love you." Let the ends of your shoulders drop. Do the same with your arms; let them relax; feel that they are fully supported by

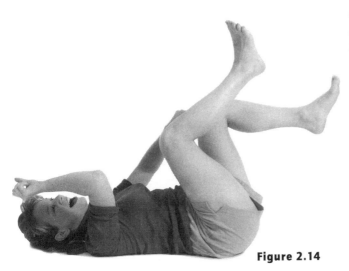

Figure 2.14

this breath of love. Rest your arms in love. Relax your wrists. Let your hands be totally relaxed in love. You're vulnerable. You don't care. You can't lose love. Breath comes in and it goes out, and love is still there. Relax your fingers, letting them curl slightly, like a baby's hand when it is asleep.

Move your attention to your chest. Be aware that you are taking a breath into your heart: "I love you." Breathe it out with love. Breathe into your lungs: "I love you." Breathe out "I love you." Now relax your entire chest. Let your breath relax in love. Become aware that this breath is love. You're not making it happen; it's happening because it loves you.

Breathe in and think of your stomach. Breathe out and say "I love you" as you relax your stomach. Relax your abdomen, thinking: "I love you. I love you the way you are." Feel the breath of love move through your hip joints. Warm, liquid, lubricating, beautiful—perfectly balanced and poised. Say "I love you" to your hips and relax them. Let the large bones in the top of your legs sink toward the floor; you don't have to hold them up. You love them. They love you. You can't lose love. Relax your legs in love. Relax your knees and ankles and think "I love you." Think to your feet "I love you." Relax your feet.

Picture yourself just simply floating; completely supported on this breath, this love. Bring your attention up to the back of your hips and the base of your spine. Open it up like a flower. Say "I love you." Don't fight it. Let it flow easily, smooth and quiet. Relax the back of your shoulder blades. Let your back get soft. Love is supporting you. "I love you, back." The back of your neck relaxes. Think to yourself, "I love you. I love you." Then you reach your brain, your hair, all soft and supported, resting in love, in breath.

Breathe in and think love. Breathe out—love is still there. Think of your brain floating in a pool of this love. Now make it totally quiet and say to yourself, "I love you." Bring your mind to your forehead and think nothing. Hold this feeling. If you feel any other thought coming in, make sure that it says "I love you." Transpose any thought to "I love you" and go back to thinking nothing. Think nothing as long as you can. Stop talking to yourself. Become silent internally.

Rest quietly like this for about 10 minutes, then slowly stretch, take a deep breath and let it out, and think about how you feel. Rest on your side or stomach for a few minutes enjoying the feeling before you get up. Move slowly back into your normal attitudes and lifestyle with new awareness.

3

THE CORE SPORTS
WARM-UP ROUTINE

At the end of a good training session I feel high, invigorated, and very hungry. As with anything else that requires so much effort, it is sometimes difficult to get started, but once I do I never regret it. During my training sessions I first work on technique and as I get more comfortable I try to empty my head of any thoughts. I try to listen to my breathing and relax my entire body. This also assists me with pain management during the long, hard workouts. For most of my training I do feel pain and exhaustion, but I try to include some easy sessions between the difficult ones.

—Dale O'Hara

I think the benefits of the asans, the whole physical part of Yoga, is so helpful in terms of the conditioning and the body strength and the breathing. And I think it gives the athlete a great edge.

—Lea Jackson

In Chapters 4–9, you will find specific suggestions for Yoga exercises (asans), breathing exercises, and other techniques to help you with the particular needs of your sport. In this chapter, we present a core routine that will benefit any athlete. The routine provides overall stretching and strengthening exercises as well as movements that increase body temperature and strengthen the respiratory system. Once you have learned the exercises, the routine will take about 10 minutes. Add to this core routine the specific suggestions found in the chapter that covers your particular sport in more detail. (Of course, feel free to practice any technique that appeals to you in any chapter.)

To get the most out of your routine, practice at a time of day when you don't feel rushed. There is no "best time of day" to practice Yoga. Some people enjoy the extra lift of practicing at dawn or in the morning; others prefer the relaxing effect of practice in early evening. If you train every day, you may be using a Yoga routine to help you warm up. The important thing is to practice a little every day—three exercises at minimum. The benefit of Yoga is cumulative; a commitment to everyday practice of even a few minutes will multiply the effects in a much shorter time than if you practice just a few days per week.

If possible, take a warm shower beforehand to help loosen your muscles; at the same time, imagine the water washing away any emotional or mental upset that may be clinging to your physical consciousness. Exercise on a blanket, a large towel, or a mat, and use it only for your Yoga routine. If you will be going directly into a sports training session afterward, you can wear regular sports attire, but don't wear shoes or socks; practice Yoga exercises barefoot. Do not practice Yoga immediately after eating a heavy meal or drinking caffeinated beverages, and never practice under the influence of alcohol or drugs.

Women should avoid Yoga exercise during the heavy days of their menstrual period, as it could cause heavy bleeding. Women who are pregnant should practice only after the first trimester and only with their doctor's permission. Specific guidelines for practicing Yoga during pregnancy are outlined in our book *The American Yoga Association Beginner's Manual* (see Resources).

When performing Yoga exercises, breathe through your nose at all times. In the previous chapter on breathing, I discussed how to focus on the steamlike sound of the breath. Continue that practice while you do Yoga asans, trying to fit the length of your breath to the movement of your body. Move slowly and deliberately. Never bounce or jerk into a position, and be careful not to strain. In Yoga, the extent of a stretch is never as important as the interplay among body, breath, and mind and the nonviolent attitude of not hurting yourself.

Try to be aware of how your body feels at all times. Check to see if you are breathing correctly and what is going through your mind. Try to stop talking to yourself. The idea is to place yourself into position with the correct breath pattern, relax any unused muscles, and bring your mind to silence. This is called the Asan Point, and you can reach this culminating point in every exercise. (A more complete discussion of the Asan Point may be found in our book *The American Yoga Association's New Yoga Challenge*. See Resources.)

You'll notice that the exercises are grouped to flow from a standing position, to kneeling on the floor, and finally to lying down. This sequencing allows you to move from one asan to the next with the least extraneous movement, enabling you to maintain a quiet, centered state of mind throughout the routine. When you add additional exercises from the chapter on your sport, you will be instructed where to add them in the core routine in order to maintain the sequential flow.

Shoulder Roll

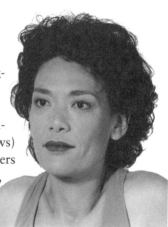

Stand with your feet parallel and arms hanging loose at your sides. Lift both shoulders up toward your ears (without bending your elbows) and rotate your shoulders in circles, first forward, then backward, at least five times in each direction (Figure 3.1). Keep your

Figure 3.1

VITAMINS AND MINERALS

Food myth: vitamin supplements boost energy levels.

With only a few exceptions (e.g., vitamin E at high altitudes and B-complex for fine motor control), vitamin and mineral supplements do not increase athletic performance in well-fed athletes. However, long-term health is affected by the athlete's diet. Many studies have noted deficiencies of calcium, iron, and zinc in athletes' diets, and increased activity means increased nutrient requirements, particularly the B-complex vitamins. Ideally, you can meet these additional requirements with the vitamins and minerals in the additional foods you eat to provide the energy your activity requires. However, if you adopt unusual or inadequate food habits, for instance to "make weight," vitamins and minerals may well be under-supplied.

If you don't consume a nutritionally sound diet, vitamin and mineral supplementation is the only means to ensure adequate intake. Deficiencies are more likely to occur with increasing training/competing activities and decreasing food intake. Vegetarian athletes who do not eat meat, fish, or poultry are unlikely to get adequate amounts of iron and zinc, too, and should consider mineral supplementation. (For best food sources for vitamins, see sidebar on page 32.)

arms and hands hanging loosely. Breathe normally throughout.

Elbow Twist

Stand with feet parallel, a few inches apart. Raise your arms to chest height and place one hand on top of the other. Breathe in completely while looking forward, then breathe out slowly as you twist toward the left, leading with your left elbow. Look around to the left so your entire upper body twists gently (Figure 3.2). Breathe in and return to the front. Breathe out and slowly twist to the right. Breathe in and return to the front. Repeat twice more to each side, alternating.

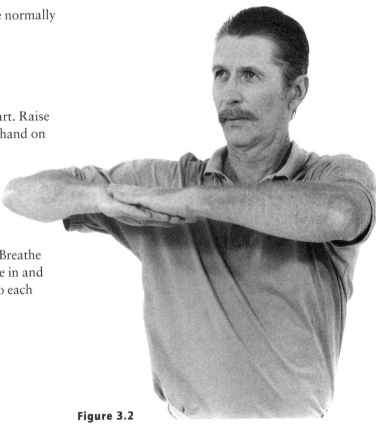

Figure 3.2

Arm Circles

Stand with feet parallel. Lift your arms straight out to the sides, fingers flexed and palms facing outward (Figure 3.3). Maintaining this position, rotate your arms first in large, slow circles and then in small, faster circles, five to eight times in each direction. Breathe normally throughout.

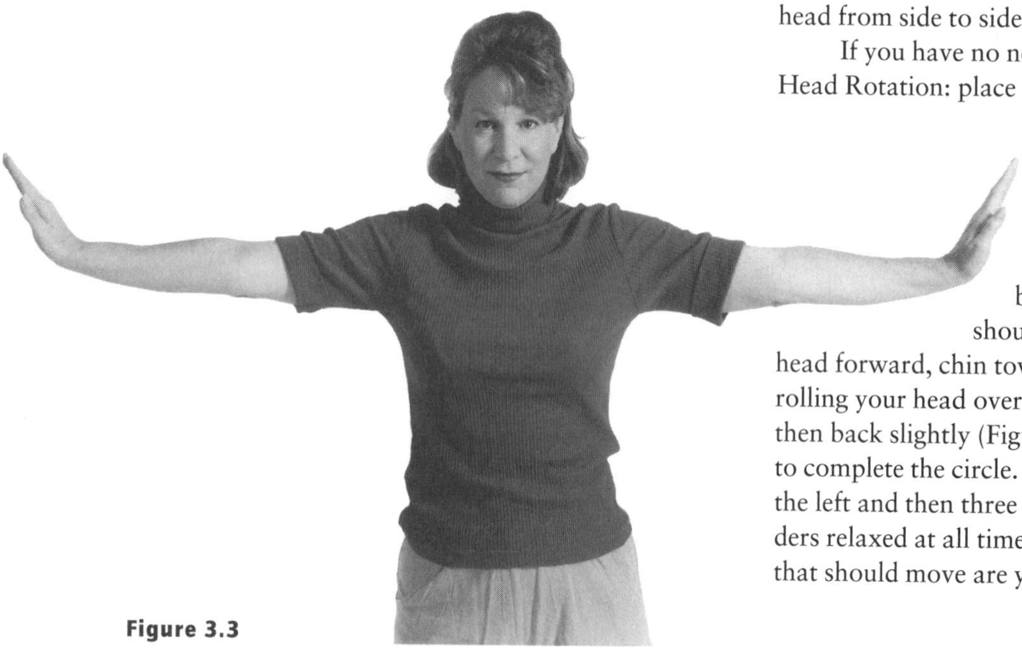

Neck Stretches

Be careful with this exercise if you have disk problems in your neck. Start by gently bending your neck to the left and slightly forward, so your chin reaches down toward your collarbone. Place your right palm on your neck to monitor the stretch (Figure 3.4). Hold for several seconds, breathing normally. Repeat on the opposite side. Release, and gently turn your head from side to side (Figure 3.5).

If you have no neck problems, you may add a Head Rotation: place your hands on your hips or let them hang straight down, and keep your shoulders relaxed. Gently bend your head to the left, bending your ear over your shoulder and being careful not to lift your shoulder up (Figure 3.6). Roll your head forward, chin toward your chest, and continue rolling your head over toward the right shoulder, then back slightly (Figure 3.7), then over to the left to complete the circle. Repeat, slowly, twice more to the left and then three times to the right. Keep shoulders relaxed at all times; the only parts of your body that should move are your head and neck.

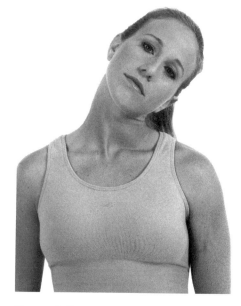

Figure 3.3

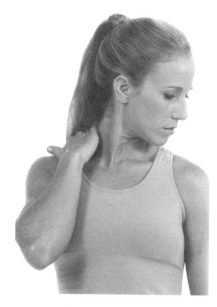

Figure 3.4

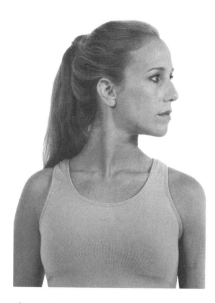

Figure 3.5

Figure 3.6

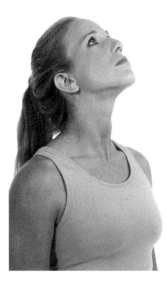

Figure 3.7

Breathe out as you bend forward from the waist, keeping your hands together and your head between your arms (Figure 3.10).

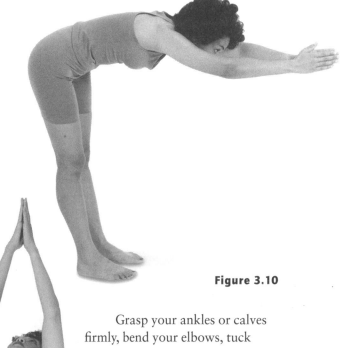

Figure 3.10

Standing Sun Pose

Stand with feet parallel. Keep your knees straight but not locked. Breathe out. Breathe in as you raise your arms in a wide circle to the sides (Figure 3.8) and overhead. Stretch and look up at your hands (Figure 3.9). Hold your breath in.

Grasp your ankles or calves firmly, bend your elbows, tuck your chin, and pull your torso toward your legs (Figure 3.11). Be sure to pull by bending your elbows instead of straining your lower back. Keep your knees straight and hold your breath out

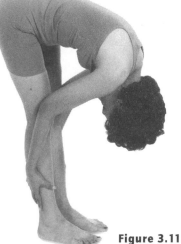

Figure 3.8   Figure 3.9   Figure 3.11

Best Food Sources of Vitamins

Follow a simple rule: grains for B-complex, fruits and vegetables for vitamins A, C, and E. Citrus, bananas, cantaloupe, and dried fruits are all excellent, and the best vegetables are always the most colorful ones. Dark green leafy vegetables such as spinach; colorful peppers; and all the members of the cruciferous family such as broccoli, cauliflower, Brussels sprouts, and cabbage; along with carrots and winter squash, are all excellent sources.

All B-complex vitamins are included in whole-grain products except for B$_{12}$, which is found in milk, eggs, and meat. Eggs also supply most of the other B-complex vitamins as do many fruits, vegetables, and meat. Vitamin D is added to milk and is formed on the skin by sunlight.

for a moment. Breathe out and slowly lower your arms to your sides. Repeat three times.

Hip Rotation

Separate your feet as wide as you can comfortably but keep your toes pointed forward. Place your hands on your hips with fingers spread on your lower back and thumbs hooked over your hips (Figure 3.13). Rotate your hips in circles several times in each direction (Figure 3.14).

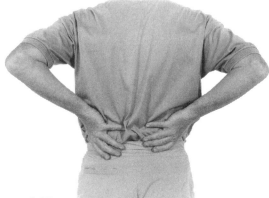

Figure 3.13

for a moment. (*Note:* if you have back or neck problems, bend only halfway down, and do not pull your torso in.)

Release and breathe in as you slowly straighten, bringing your arms in a wide circle to the sides (Figure 3.12) and over your head again. Look up and stretch as in Figure 3.9. Hold your breath in

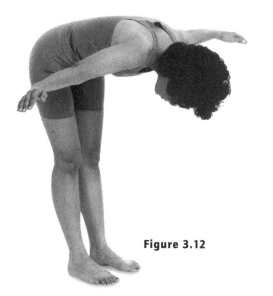

Figure 3.12

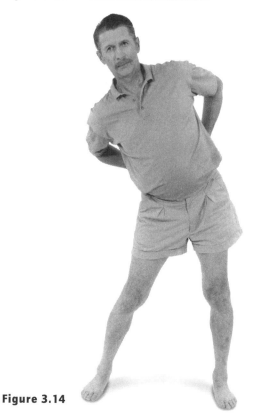

Figure 3.14

Side Triangle

With feet still separated, toes pointed forward, breathe in completely, arms outstretched (Figure 3.15), then breathe out and bend sideways toward the right, sliding your right hand down your right leg. Bring your left arm up and over your head, keeping it as straight as possible; stretch from your waist (Figure 3.16). Look at a spot on the wall straight in front of you. Hold your breath out. Breathe in as you return to the starting position. Repeat three times to each side, alternating.

Twisting Triangle

With feet still separated, breathe in completely, keep arms outstretched (Figure 3.17), then breathe out as you bend toward your left leg. Grasp the outside of your left leg with your right hand and pull gently as you twist your torso left, bringing your left arm straight up toward the ceiling. Make a loose fist with your upraised hand and look at your left thumb (Figure 3.18). Hold your breath out for a moment.

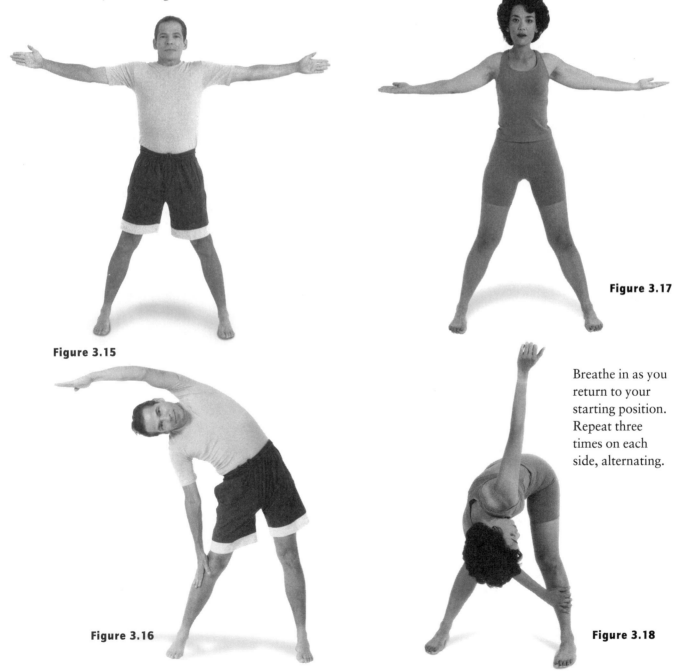

Figure 3.17

Figure 3.15

Breathe in as you return to your starting position. Repeat three times on each side, alternating.

Figure 3.16

Figure 3.18

Cat Breath

Come down to the floor on your hands and knees. Breathe in as you arch your back and look up toward the ceiling (Figure 3.19). Hold your breath in. Breathe out as you round your back, tuck your chin into your chest, pull in and up on your stomach, and contract your rectal muscles (Figure 3.20). Hold your breath out. Repeat three times.

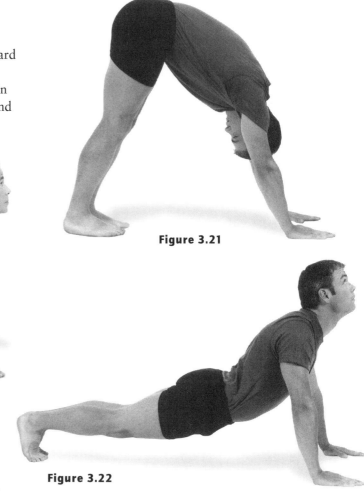

Figure 3.21

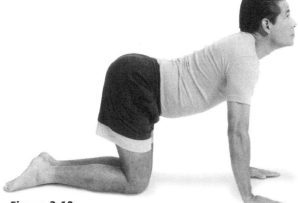

Figure 3.19

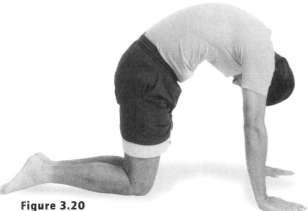

Figure 3.20

Cobra V-Raise

Straighten your legs and walk your hands out to the V position (Figure 3.21). Tuck your head, push your heels to the floor, and breathe out. Hold your breath out for a moment.

Breathe in as you lower your hips toward the floor and arch your back, keeping your arms and legs

Figure 3.22

straight (supporting yourself only on hands and feet). Look up toward the ceiling (Figure 3.22). Hold your breath in for a moment. Repeat three times.

Baby Pose

Kneel and sit on your feet. Bend forward, keeping your hips on your feet, so your forehead or the top of your head rests on the floor. Bring your arms to your sides and let your elbows fall outward slightly so that your shoulders relax completely (Figure 3.23). Breathe naturally and relax your entire body. Hold for as long as you comfortably can. If you cannot bend completely forward while keeping your hips on your feet due to a large midsection or stiff knees or hips, just bend as far forward as you can. It's more important to try to keep your hips on your heels than to rest your head on the floor.

If you have high blood pressure, or if placing your head lower than your heart is uncomfortable, rest your head on folded arms (Figure 3.24), but try to keep your hips on your feet.

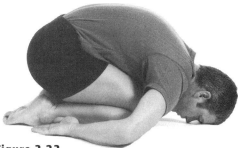

Figure 3.23

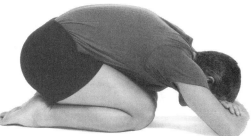

Figure 3.24

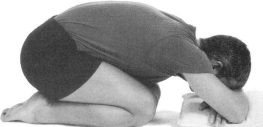

Figure 3.25

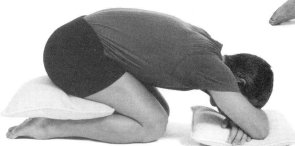

Figure 3.26

If your knees or hips are too stiff for this position, place a pillow under your arms to release some of the pressure (Figure 3.25). You can also add a pillow under your hips (Figure 3.26).

Cobra Pose

Stretch forward so that you are lying on your stomach. Bring your hands close in to your body under your armpits, with elbows raised, and your forehead to the floor (Figure 3.27). Breathe out. Breathe in as you first curl your head back, then lift your chest off the floor, then your stomach, using your back muscles more than your arms. Keep your eyes focused between your eyebrows (Figure 3.28). Hold your breath in for a moment.

Breathe out as you curl down in reverse: stomach first, then chest, then head, bringing your forehead back to the floor. Repeat three times.

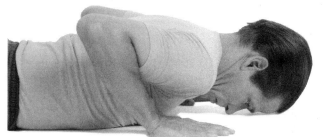

Figure 3.27

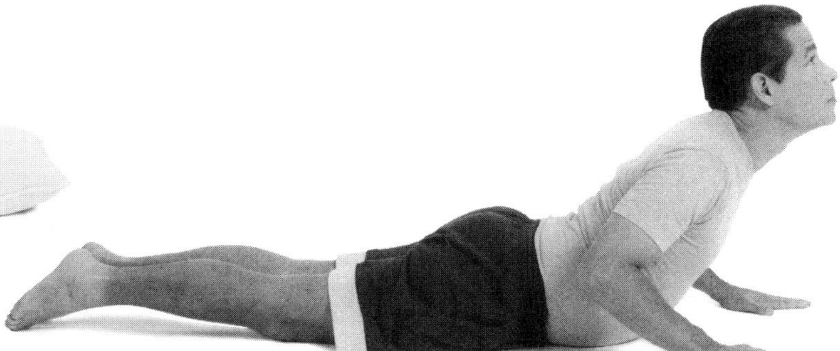

Figure 3.28

Knee Squeeze

Lie on your back with arms overhead and legs together (Figure 3.29). Breathe out completely. Breathe in as you bend your left knee and grasp it with both hands, bringing it in toward your chest, then squeeze your knee to your chest and lift your forehead up toward your knee (Figure 3.30). Hold your breath in for a moment. Relax and breathe out as you lower your head, arms, and legs down to the floor back to your starting position. Repeat with the left leg, then twice more on each side, alternating.

Rest a moment, then do the same movement with both legs at the same time. Hold your breath in as you try to touch your forehead to your knees (Figure 3.31). Breathe out and relax back to your starting position. Repeat three times.

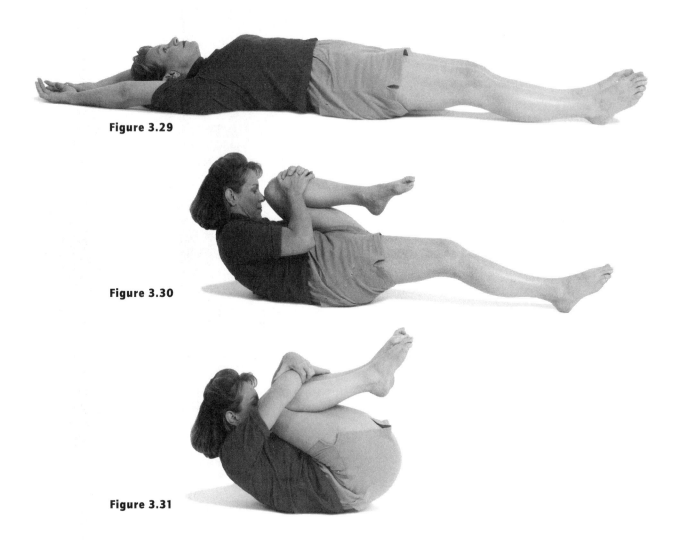

Figure 3.29

Figure 3.30

Figure 3.31

4

TARGET SPORTS

Archery, Golf, Long Jump, High Jump, Baseball/Softball, Volleyball, and Basketball

Before every shot I take a complete breath to focus my attention on the task at hand, to bring my awareness into the moment, and to rest in the silence of the spiritual body. I carefully observe the situation, conditions, my feelings, emotions, and level of play. I carefully consider my options of play, remembering that the conservative play is almost always the smart play. I then creatively and intuitively, while relying on the spiritual body, decide on the shot to play. I see it, I feel it, and I trust it. I select the club. While holding it in my hands I transmit the feel of that great shot I've decided upon directly into the club, all the way into the sweet spot on the club face. I then take a practice swing, eyes closed, thinking only of the feel of that great shot I've decided upon, hit directly on the sweet spot of the club. As I finish the swing, I open my eyes and see the practice shot go

exactly where I want it to go. I precisely line up the shot. Then, without fear of contrary results, I take dead aim with one-pointed concentration to hit the shot I've decided upon, and by so doing, offer the fruit of my actions to the divine. I see it, I feel it, I trust it. I swing and hit the shot. After each shot, I carefully observe the results. I evaluate, analyze, integrate, and learn from the results, but I do not judge myself over the results because I am not my golfing performance. Golf is Yoga for me. I stay equanimous, balanced, and centered, and at all times, I breathe.

—DAVID TIPTON

Ninety percent of hitting is mental. The other half is physical.

—YOGI BERRA

The crucial moment in target sports is the moment of release: when the arrow leaves your bow, when your body leaves the ground in the long or high jump, when you swing the bat toward the onrushing ball, when you let go of the ball, or when you send your putt toward the cup. In all cases the similarity is that you loft your effort into an area where the physical is no longer in control. That moment of release in space-time is unknowable. The mind goes silent; all concentration is on the release.

Of course, your physical preparation and the manner in which you use your physical body to approach the point of release are part of the ability to achieve the distance or hit the target, but despite rigorous training of the physical, the outcome of the release cannot be predicted. Some days you can hit the target easily, and some days you can't. Some throws are better than others; jumpers have good days and bad; basketball players sometimes make all their foul shots and sometimes cannot; and once in a great while golfers hit a hole in one. Most athletes feel that proper physical training alone is the answer to being able always to achieve the perfect effort, and often the workout of the physical body becomes very stressful in order to produce a predictable result. In spite of this, results still vary, and a great many of the surprising differences are due to the emotional involvement of the athlete.

The awareness of the inner body, the soul of the athlete, is represented in the modern Olympiad. Great importance is given to the ideal of maintenance of purity and clear purpose in the athlete that allows the inner emotional force of the body to show its strength in sport. When the responsibility for all result is placed on the physical body alone, the demand often breaks the athlete down. The physical body must be able to call on the equal support of the emotional body that lies within.

In ancient times, sports were worshiped as a divine display of the emotional/spiritual/power body that supports the physical body in the form of breath. Breath was considered the source of life. Although it is without physical form, breath is able to show its presence and power in the athletic trials of sport. Breath is the bridge that connects the two bodies. Your outer physical self and your inner emotional/spiritual/power being are pulled together for the final release. This release to fly rests on the breath, which supports your effort into the unknown, that point of release where your effort is projected into space, free of the physical.

USING THE BREATH TO JUMP

The long jump and the high jump really epitomize the old Greek proverb "Nothing is so bold as a blind horse." Pulling together all your strength and hurling yourself into the air takes courage—and extreme confidence. You hope you will be able to land correctly, but you can't be sure.

This training can be greatly enhanced by fantasy meditative exercise. Before the actual jump begins, sit or lie quietly in silence with your eyes closed. Carefully visualize each step leading up to your jump. When you reach your lift-off point, mentally fantasize your breath forming a large ball within your solar plexus. Then begin your leap with the visualized picture of yourself being lifted by this ball of breath. When you reach the peak of your lift, let the air out of the ball as you land *where* you wish, and *how* you wish.

Practice this exercise three times mentally before you perform the actual jump. The exercise will take you only four or five minutes, and it will help you perform with a harmonious composure that will give you better distance and protect you from injury. As you gain familiarity with the exercise, you can achieve the same results with the remembrance of the visionary experience in a few moments of concentration before your leap. It will become automatic.

Yoga training's emphasis on bridging the outer and inner bodies presents another great benefit to target athletes due to their sports' dependence on precise fine motor control. Through Yoga training, you can learn to approach athletic practice and performance with a calm, balanced attitude of confidence that, once learned, is very difficult to lose. The result is a constant, cool, and calculated state of mind that gives you the best chance of achieving your goal.

Lately, in the process of writing this book, the most interesting part of my conversations with athletes occurs when I ask them what they think about just before they make their kick, shot, or throw. The answer is always "Nothing. If I think about anything my effort is not the best. If I can move to no thought just as I try for the supreme effort, I have the best chance to succeed."

When I probe further, asking "Well, if you don't think about what you are doing, how do you know you will do your best?" their answer is always the same: "I don't know. I have to wait and see."

> *I practice what's called "instinctive shooting." You don't think how many yards it is. You look at the target and you concentrate and your mind takes over your left arm and you shoot. And after you get good, you hit the target. There is nothing to aim with. Your arm will find the target without thinking about it. When I go up to full draw, I don't stay up more than four seconds. The longer you stay up, you get in trouble because you start thinking about other things. We all have the basic talent to shoot without the equipment. The mind takes over. And something tells you when your arm is right.*
>
> —George Nodaros, archer

The Sport Routines

Target sports can be greatly helped by the regular practice of focusing techniques. For example, the Eye Exercise, included in the routine for Archery, on page 42, will be helpful for any other target sport as well. Balancing exercises are also key for developing concentration, steadiness, and intuition. For best results, always include a few minutes of breathing and meditation in your daily Yogic routine.

Archery

Since archery is a one-sided sport (see Chapter 5), archers need to balance both sides of the body. "Instinctive shooting" can be sharpened by training in concentration and steadiness through breathing techniques and meditation. Yoga exercises will improve overall flexibility and strengthen the lower back to provide support for the strong upper body that archers develop.

Due to the extreme upper-body strength required for this sport, archers can experience lower back pain. The best way to prevent these injuries is through strengthening of the lower back and abdominal muscles.

Modify your core routine as follows:

Tree Pose

Add this exercise between the Standing Sun Pose and the Hip Rotation (pages 31–32). From a standing position, lift your right foot and place it on the inside of your left thigh (Figure 4.1). Relax the leg to help hold your foot in position. Bare feet will also help. If you feel unsteady, hold on to a sturdy chair. Steady yourself by gazing at one spot on the wall or floor

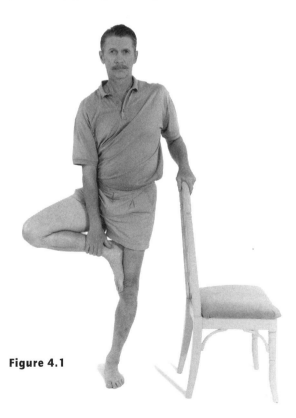

Figure 4.1

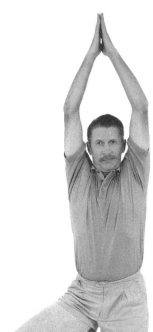

Figure 4.2

Arm and Leg Balance

Add this exercise between the Cat Breath and the Cobra V-Raise (page 34). Start on your hands and knees. Breathe out completely, then breathe in as you lift your left arm and right leg (opposites) parallel to the floor (Figure 4.4). Stare at one spot and hold your breath in for a moment. Breathe out, release, and repeat with the opposite arm and leg. Repeat three times on each side.

    Variation: lift the arm and leg on the same side of the body (Figure 4.5).

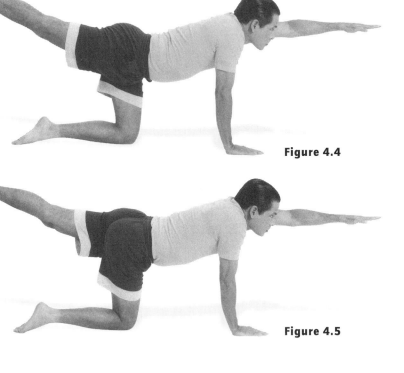

Figure 4.4

Figure 4.5

without bending your neck. Breathe in as you raise your arms slowly over your head, straighten your arms, and place your palms together (Figure 4.2). Hold your breath in for a moment. Breathe out and bring your arms and leg down slowly. Repeat on the opposite side.

    If you are limber enough, you may place your foot on top of your thigh for this exercise (Figure 4.3).

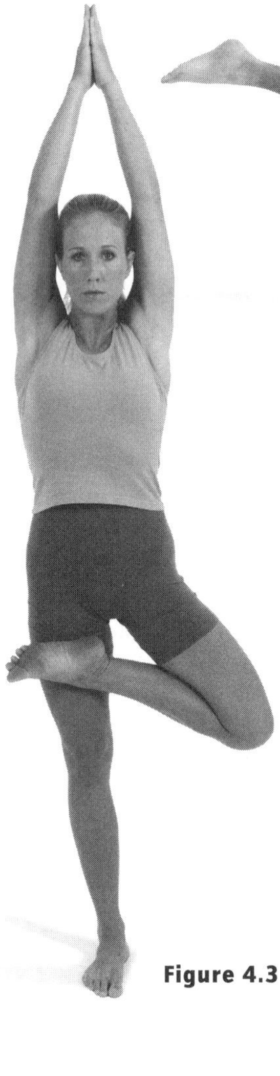

Figure 4.3

Plank Pose (pictured, page 45)

Add the next three exercises between the Baby Pose and the Cobra Pose (pages 34–35). From a hands-and-knees position, straighten your legs out behind you, supporting yourself on your hands. Raise your hips and lower your shoulders until your body is in a straight line supported on your hands and feet. Shift your weight to your right arm and breathe in as you lift your left arm straight in front of you. Focus your gaze on your outstretched hand. Hold your breath in for a moment. Breathe out and release.

    Still supporting yourself on your right arm, breathe in as you bring your left arm to the side and up toward the ceiling. This will twist your body to the left as well. Look up toward your hand. Hold your breath in for a moment. Breathe out, bring your left hand down to the floor, and repeat the sequence on the opposite side. Then rest lying on your stomach.

Side Stretch

Sit up in a comfortable cross-legged position. Breathe in, then breathe out as you lean to the right and stretch your left arm up over your head and toward the right, stretching the entire left side of your torso (Figure 4.6). Hold your breath out for a moment. Breathe in as you release, then repeat on the opposite side.

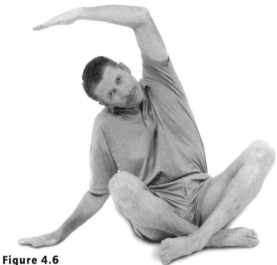

Figure 4.6

Back Strengthener Series
(pictured, pages 58–60)

Stretch your arms on the floor over your head and place your forehead on the floor. Breathe out. Breathe in as you lift your arms, legs, and head, looking up through your forehead. (This exercise is also called the Boat Pose.) Hold your breath in for a moment.

Breathe out and release, bringing both arms straight out to the sides, palms down, and forehead to the floor. Rest a moment, then breathe in as you lift your arms, legs, and head, looking up through your forehead. Hold your breath in for a moment.

Breathe out and release, bringing your arms down to your sides. Rest a moment, then breathe in as you lift your arms, legs, and head, looking up through your forehead. Hold your breath in for a moment.

Breathe out and release, bringing your arms behind your back with your fingers clasped. Rest a moment, then breathe in as you lift your arms, legs, and head, pressing your palms together and straightening your arms as much as possible so your shoulder blades are squeezed together and your arms stretch away from your body. Look up through your forehead. Hold your breath in for a moment.

Breathe out and release, bending your knees and grasping your feet with both hands. Rest a moment with your forehead to the floor, then breathe in as you lift, pulling up on your feet so you balance on your stomach. (This position is also called the Bow Pose.) Look up through your forehead. Hold your breath in for a moment. Breathe out and release. Rest on your stomach.

Alternate Toe Touch

Add the next four exercises after the Knee Squeeze (page 36). Lie on your back with your arms overhead and your legs together (Figure 4.7). Breathe out. Breathe in as you lift your right arm and left leg and reach for your big toe (Figure 4.8). If you can, grasp the toe with your thumb and forefinger. (If you are very limber, you can reach around your big toe with your hand, as in the Alternate Seated Sun Pose, page 87, Figures 6.13–6.17). Another way to stretch into this position is to first bend the left knee, grasp the toe, and carefully straighten the leg as far as you can without strain. Repeat once on each side.

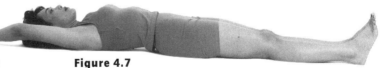

Figure 4.7

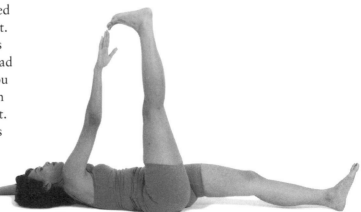

Figure 4.8

Variation: lift arm and leg on the same side of the body (Figure 4.9).

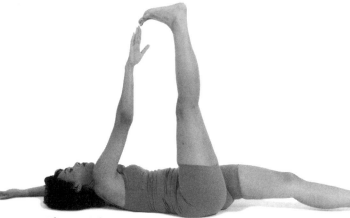

Figure 4.9

Hand-Limbering Exercises
(pictured, page 56)
Repeat each of the following movements several times. Spread your fingers wide apart, then make fists. Press the fingers of one hand back using the opposite hand. Repeat on the opposite side. Make a "steeple" with your fingers and press the fingers together.

Humming Breath
Sit up in a comfortable position, either cross-legged or sitting on your feet, or sit on the edge of a chair with your hands on your knees. Breathe in completely just as you would in the Complete Breath, described on page 20. Now breathe out with an audible *hummmm* sound, making the tone steady and loud until your breath is gone—just like the sound of a bumblebee. Let the sound vibrate in your throat, and keep pushing with your belly muscles so that the sound doesn't trail off at the end. Try to keep the sound steady. Repeat several times.

Eye Exercise
Hold a pencil (or just your thumb) out at arm's length (Figure 4.10). Focus your eyes on the tip of the pencil. Now shift your focus to an object at the far end of the room, for example a lamp or picture. Shift your focus back and forth from the pencil to the far wall a few more times. Don't strain. Close your eyes and relax.

When I can strike that balance of sharp play, the confidence to continue, and a balanced outlook, I can score very well and the game feels "easy" to play. Many great golfers talk and write about playing in the "zone," where golf feels much simpler to play than normal and good shots seem to come with little effort. Some refer to this as being able to get out of your own way to play your best. This feeling is wonderful. I am very interested in being able to put myself in my zone at will, and not just wait for it to happen on its own. To do this, however, seems to require a talented walk across a razor's edge. It seems that the harder one tries to play well or bring on that feeling, the more elusive it can be. There seems to be an element of having to let go of trying to force that state of mind and trust it to come, in order to be able to bring that feeling into play more often. I really enjoy this pursuit. When I am succeeding at it, it feels like I am giving it, not getting it.

—David Tipton

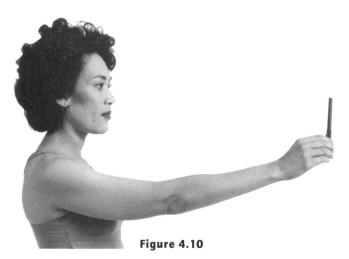

Figure 4.10

Golf

Golf requires a strong back, good concentration, and spinal flexibility. Because golf is a one-sided game, the body tends to become imbalanced over time. Yoga can help balance both sides of the body and provide overall flexibility training. The breathing techniques and meditation training of Yoga can improve focus and sharpen a player's concentration.

Muscles on the nondominant side of the body are particularly vulnerable to strain because of the extreme twisting motion of the golf swing. The best way to prevent these injuries is thorough warm-up and an all-around program of flexibility and strength exercises.

Modify your core routine as follows:

Alternate Triangle

Add this exercise between the Hip Rotation and the Side Triangle (pages 32–33). Maintain the Hip Rotation position with legs spread. Breathe in and stretch your arms out to the sides (Figure 4.11), then breathe out as you bend toward your right leg. Remember to keep your knees straight but not locked. Holding your breath out for a moment, grasp your right ankle firmly with both hands, bend your elbows, and pull gently, keeping your knees straight and tucking your

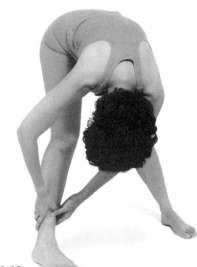

Figure 4.12

chin into your chest (Figure 4.12). Breathe in as you return to the starting position. Repeat three times to each leg, alternating.

T Pose (pictured, page 48)

Add the next two exercises between the Twisting Triangle and the Cat Breath (pages 33–34). When you are first learning this position, stand three to four feet from a chair or other support. Lean forward and hold on to the support with both hands. Lift your left leg in back as high as you can, ideally, parallel to the floor. Alternatively, brace yourself with both hands on the knee of your supporting leg. Keep your right (supporting) leg straight. Your torso and left leg should be in a straight line parallel to the floor. Keep your neck straight, breathe naturally, and look at a spot on the floor.

When you feel steady, release your grip on the support and place your palms together, pushing your arms out parallel to the floor. Relax your breath. Look forward at your hands. Lower your leg and return to a standing position. Rest until your breath returns to normal. Repeat on the opposite side.

Dancer Pose and Extension

From a standing position, bend your left leg back and grasp your left foot with your right hand (Figure 4.13). Throughout the exercise, steady yourself by fixing your gaze on one spot on the wall in front of you. Slowly move into the completed Dancer Pose by raising your left arm straight up toward the ceiling and pulling your lifted leg up and back as far as possible without strain (Figure 4.14). Keep your right

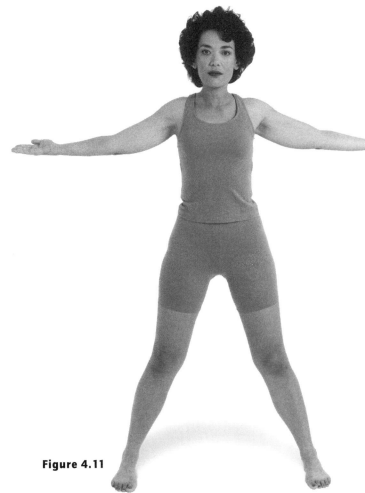

Figure 4.11

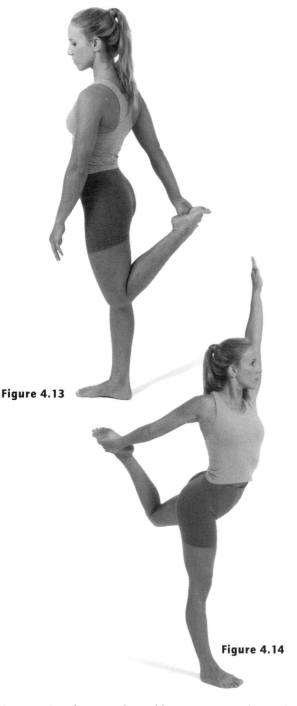

Figure 4.13

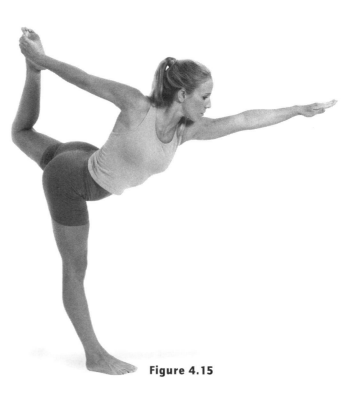

Figure 4.15

Figure 4.14

Cat Variation

Add this exercise between the Cat Breath and the Cobra V-Raise (page 34). This sequence is done with a strong, steady breath pattern. On hands and knees, start by breathing in. Breathe out strongly as you round your back up and forward and bring your right knee to your forehead (Figure 4.16).

Breathe in briefly as you release that position and breathe out again strongly as you go into the next position. Straighten and lift your right leg in back, bend your elbows, and arch your back so your chin reaches toward the floor (Figure 4.17). Breathe in briefly as you release that position and breathe out as you go back to the first position (Figure 4.16) for the next repetition. Repeat three to six times on each side, slowly.

(supporting) leg straight and keep your gaze focused on one spot. Breathe in and hold your breath in for a moment.

Maintaining your gaze, slowly breathe out and lower your body into the extended position (Figure 4.15). Keep your lifted leg as far up and back as possible. Your left arm extends straight ahead. Your supporting leg remains straight. Stare at one spot for balance. Don't strain. Hold for a moment, then breathe in, come back to a standing position, and switch sides.

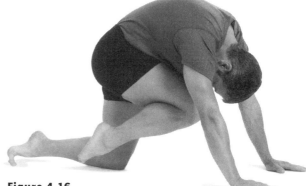

Figure 4.16

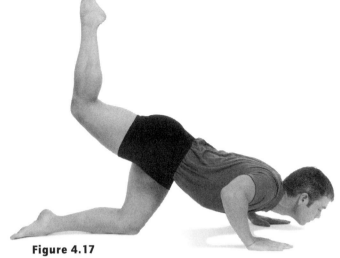

Figure 4.17

Bow Variation (pictured, pages 53–54)

Add this exercise between the Cobra V-Raise and the Baby Pose (pages 34–35). Start on your hands and knees. Reach back with your left hand and grasp your right foot. Stare at one spot on the wall or floor for balance as you breathe in and lift your foot up and away from your body as far as possible. Hold your breath in for a moment. Breathe out, release slowly, and switch sides. Repeat three times on each side.

Spine Twist (pictured, pages 51–52)

Add the next two exercises between the Baby Pose and the Cobra Pose (pages 34–35). Sit up with both legs bent in front of you. Bend your left knee and lay it on the floor with your left foot under your right knee. Pick up your right foot and carry it across your left knee. Pull your left foot in close to your body.

Turn toward the right and bring your left arm over your right knee. With your left elbow, press your right knee back as far as it will comfortably go, then straighten your left arm and grasp the right big toe. If you can't reach your toe, grasp your ankle or knee instead.

Bring your right hand close in to your body, fingers pointed in, and straighten your arm. Straighten your back, breathe in looking forward, then breathe out as you twist toward the right as far as you can without straining. Look at a spot on the wall just above eye level. Hold your breath out for a moment.

Release, and repeat on the opposite side.

Variation: for a less strenuous pose, keep the left leg outstretched.

Plank Pose

From a hands-and-knees position, straighten your legs out behind you, supporting yourself on your hands. Raise your hips and lower your shoulders until your body is in a straight line supported on your hands and feet (Figure 4.18). Shift your weight to your right arm and breathe in as you lift your left arm straight in front of you (Figure 4.19). Focus your gaze on your outstretched hand. Hold your breath in for a moment. Breathe out and release.

Still supporting yourself on your right arm, breathe in as you bring your left arm to the side and up toward the ceiling (Figure 4.20). This will twist your body to the left as well. Look up toward your hand. Hold your breath in for a moment. Breathe out, bring your left hand down to the floor, and repeat the sequence on the opposite side. The rest lying on your stomach.

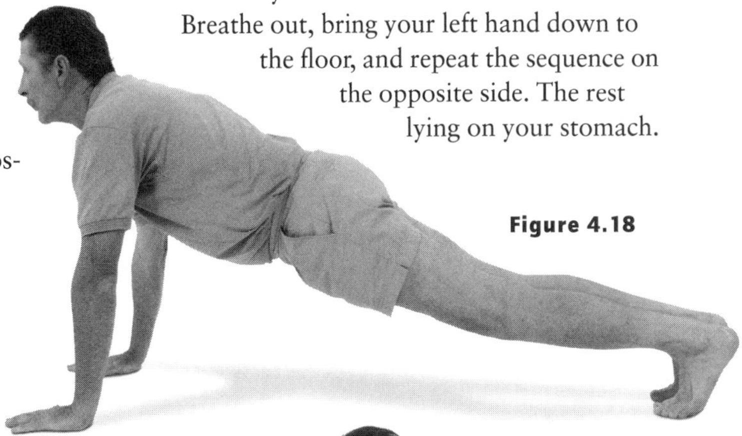

Figure 4.18

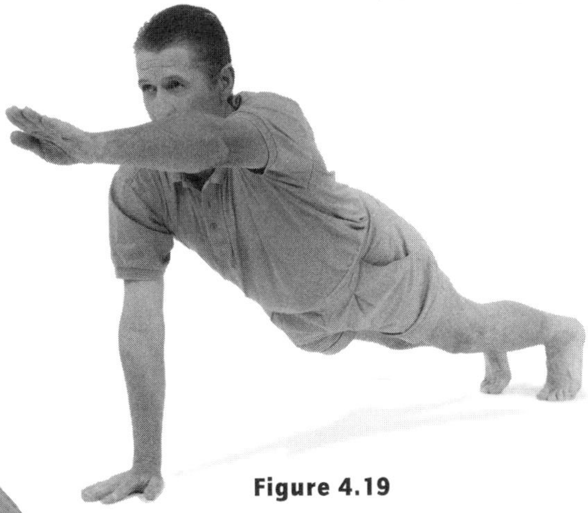

Figure 4.19

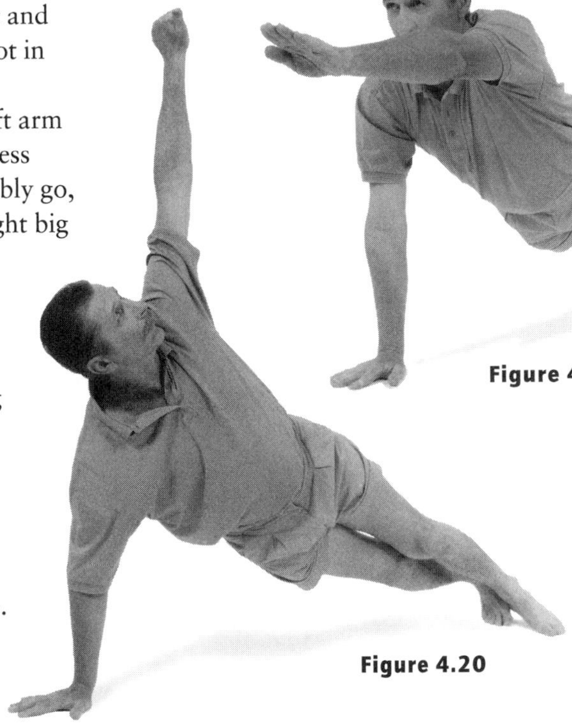

Figure 4.20

Back Strengthener Series
(pictured, pages 58–60)

Add this exercise between the Cobra Pose and the Knee Squeeze (pages 35–36). Stretch your arms on the floor over your head and place your forehead on the floor. Breathe out. Breathe in as you lift your arms, legs, and head, looking up through your forehead. (This exercise is also called the Boat Pose.) Hold your breath in for a moment.

Breathe out and release, bringing both arms straight out to the sides, palms down, and forehead to the floor. Rest a moment, then breathe in as you lift your arms, legs, and head, looking up through your forehead. Hold your breath in for a moment.

Breathe out and release, bringing your arms down to your sides. Rest a moment, then breathe in as you lift your arms, legs, and head, looking up through your forehead. Hold your breath in for a moment.

Breathe out and release, bringing your arms behind your back with your fingers clasped. Rest a moment, then breathe in as you lift your arms, legs, and head, pressing your palms together and straightening your arms as much as possible so your shoulder blades are squeezed together and your arms stretch away from your body. Look up through your forehead. Hold your breath in for a moment.

Breathe out and release, bending your knees and grasping your feet with both hands. Rest a moment with your forehead to the floor, then breathe in as you lift, pulling up on your feet so you balance on your stomach. (This position is also called the Bow Pose.) Look up through your forehead. Hold your breath in for a moment. Breathe out and release. Rest on your stomach.

Alternate Toe Touch
(pictured, page 41)

Add the next two exercises after the Knee Squeeze (page 36). Lie on your back with your arms overhead and your legs together. Breathe out. Breathe in as you lift your right arm and left leg and reach for your big toe. If you can, grasp the toe with your thumb and forefinger. (If you are very limber, you can reach around your big toe with your hand, as in the Alternate Seated Sun Pose, page 143, Figure 8.14.) Another way to stretch into this position is to first bend the left knee, grasp the toe, and carefully straighten the leg as far as you can without strain. Repeat once on each side.

Humming Breath

Sit up in a comfortable position, either cross-legged or sitting on your feet, or sit on the edge of a chair with your hands on your knees. Breathe in completely just as you would in the Complete Breath, described on page 20. Now breathe out with an audible *hummmm* sound, making the tone steady and loud until your breath is gone—just like the sound of a bumblebee. Let the sound vibrate in your throat, and keep pushing with your belly muscles so that the sound doesn't trail off at the end. Try to keep the sound steady. Repeat several times.

DO YOU HAVE A CARBOHYDRATE COMPLEX? STARCHES VS. SUGAR

Carbohydrates can be either simple (sugar) or complex (starch). Starches are ideal for sustaining blood glucose (increasing stamina) and for building glycogen reserves, while sugar may cause low blood sugar by triggering excess insulin production. Starch is less apt to produce this response. Many athletes depend on sugar to stave off hunger—but they wouldn't be hungry if their diet were richer in starchy foods. Food starches are better sources for fuel, too, because they do not contain empty calories, and instead are always loaded with essential vitamins and minerals. Since complex carbohydrates sustain blood sugar, they are the best choice for low-calorie restricted diets, too. (For more on carbohydrates, see sidebars on pages 14 and 18.)

Long Jump/High Jump

These events require great flexibility in the hips and legs, and a good sense of balance and timing. There will be some imbalance in the body, as the same leg is usually used to push off, and the other to lead into the jump. Yoga exercises will thoroughly stretch out leg and back muscles to avoid injury, balance both

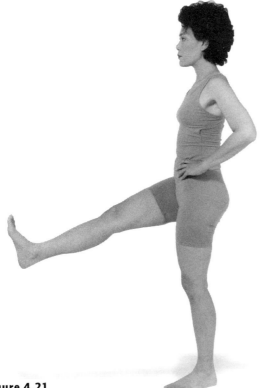

Figure 4.21

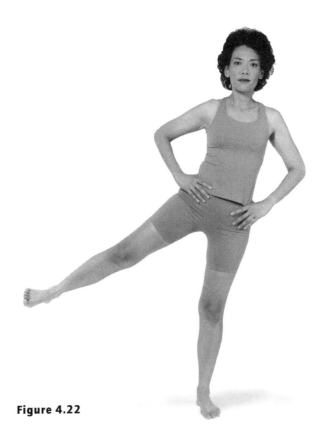

Figure 4.22

sides of the body, and strengthen the lower back; you can use a fantasy exercise to focus your imagination and see yourself accomplishing the jump. Practice fantasy using your nondominant leg to push off, then return to your dominant side and fantasize the same movement.

Athletes involved in these events often experience strains in leg muscles and groin pulls. The best way to prevent these injuries is to stretch the leg muscles in all directions, and to strengthen the knees and lower body.

Modify your core routine as follows:

Leg Raises

Add the next two exercises between the Neck Stretches and the Standing Sun Pose (pages 30–32). Stand straight with both hands on your hips. (If you feel unsteady, you can hold on to a chair with your right hand.) Breathe out completely. Breathe in as you lift your right leg straight up in front as high as possible without bending your knee or straining (Figure 4.21). Hold the position and your breath for a moment. Breathe out and lower your leg. Breathe in and lift your right leg straight out to the side as far as possible without straining (Figure 4.22). Hold the position and your breath for a moment. Breathe out and lower your leg. Breathe in and lift your right leg straight out in back as far as possible without bending your knee (Figure 4.23). Hold the position and your breath for a moment. Breathe out and lower your leg. Repeat with your left leg.

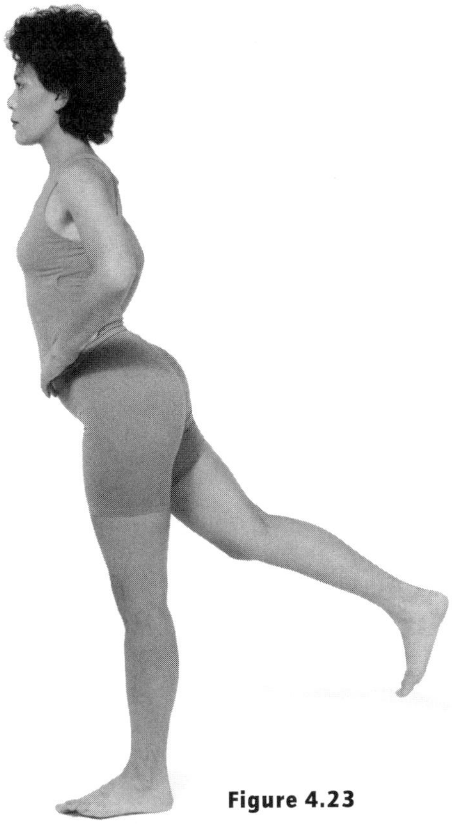

Figure 4.23

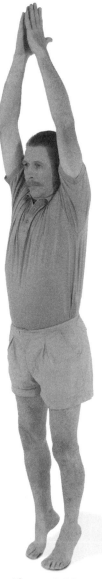

Figure 4.24

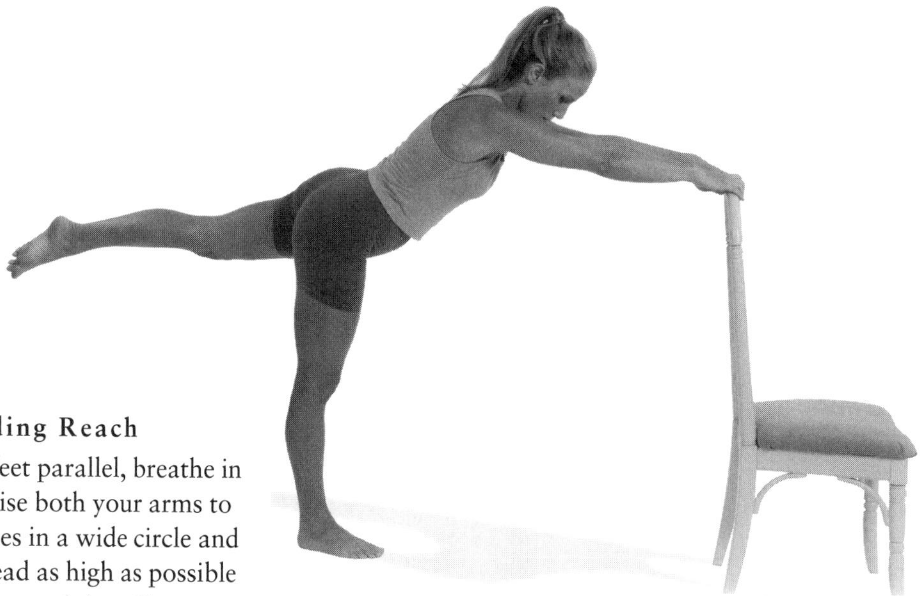

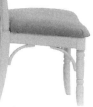

Figure 4.25

Standing Reach

With feet parallel, breathe in and raise both your arms to the sides in a wide circle and overhead as high as possible without straining. Come up on your toes and stretch up toward the ceiling (Figure 4.24). Hold your breath in for a moment. Breathe out as you slowly lower your arms to your sides. Relax. Repeat twice more.

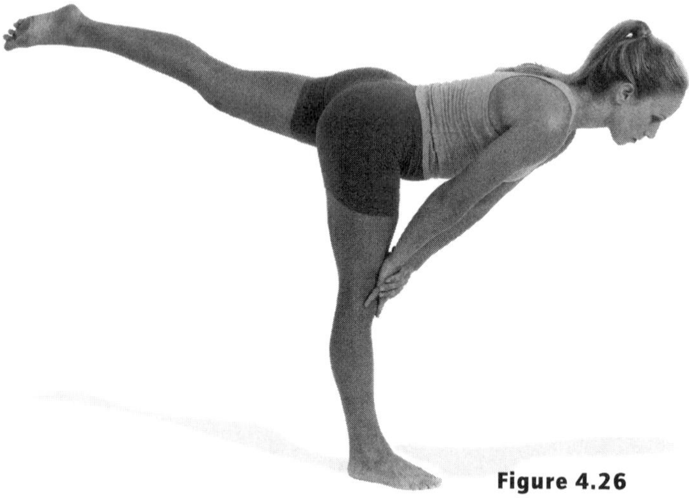

T Pose

Add the next four exercises between the Standing Sun Pose and the Hip Rotation (pages 31–32). When you are first learning this position, stand three to four feet from a chair or other support. Lean forward and hold on to the support with both hands. Lift your left leg in back as high as you can (Figure 4.25), ideally, parallel to the floor. Alternatively, brace yourself with both hands on the knee of your supporting leg (Figure 4.26). Keep your right (supporting) leg straight. Your torso and left leg should be in a straight line parallel to the floor. Keep your neck straight, breathe naturally, and look at a spot on the floor.

Figure 4.26

When you feel steady, release your grip on the support and place your palms together, pushing your arms out parallel to the floor (Figure 4.27). Relax your breath. Look forward at your hands. Lower your leg and return to a standing position. Rest until your breath returns to normal. Repeat on the opposite side.

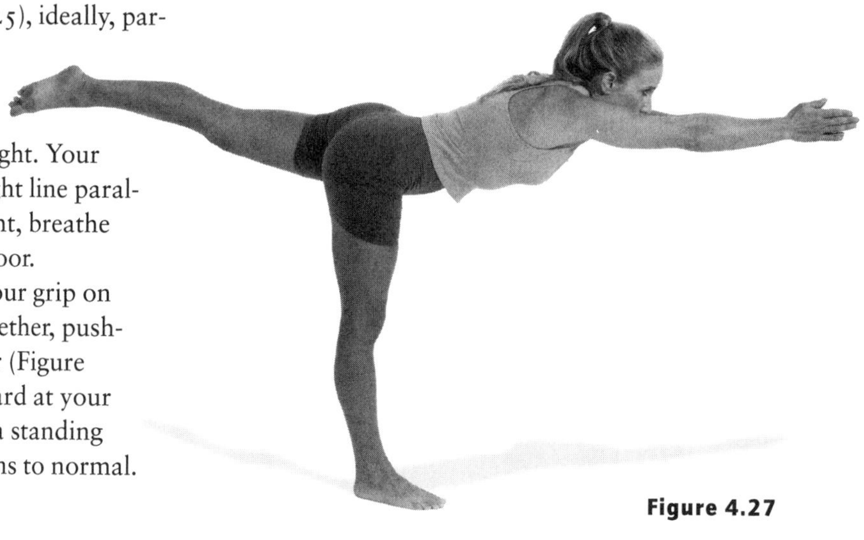

Figure 4.27

Warrior Pose

When you are strong enough, you can perform this exercise immediately after the T Pose on one side, then repeat both exercises on the opposite side.

Place both hands on your right knee and lift your left leg straight in back. Bend your right knee and let your torso rest on your right thigh as you slide your hands down to support either side of your right ankle (Figures 4.28 and 4.29). Keep your left leg high in back. Tuck your head. Breathe out and hold your breath out for a moment. Breathe in, slowly release, and repeat on the opposite side.

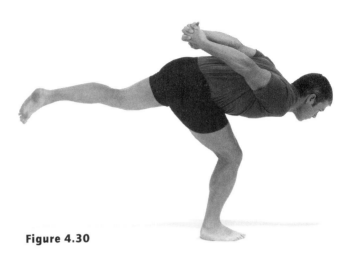

Figure 4.30

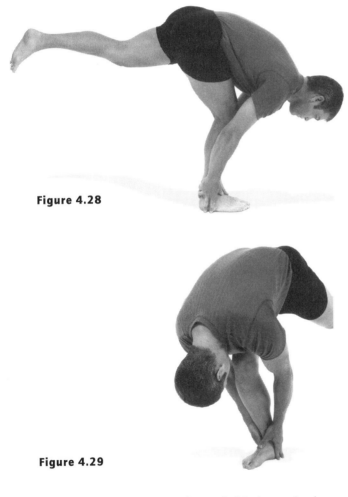

Figure 4.28

Figure 4.29

Variation: lace your fingers behind your back. If you can, lock your elbows, squeezing your shoulder blades together. Lift one leg as high as possible, bend your supporting leg, rest your chest on your thigh if possible, and lift your arms away from your back (Figure 4.30). Breathe out and hold for a moment. Release and switch sides.

Rest in a Standing Position

Feet should be parallel, a few inches apart. Let your arms rest at your sides. Close your eyes. Let your breath return to normal.

Dancer Pose and Extension
(pictured, page 44)

From a standing position, bend your left leg back and grasp your left foot with your right hand. Throughout the exercise, steady yourself by fixing your gaze on one spot on the wall in front of you. Slowly move into the completed Dancer Pose by raising your left arm straight up toward the ceiling and pulling your lifted leg up and back as far as possible without strain (as shown in Figure 4.14). Keep your right (supporting) leg straight and keep your gaze focused on one spot. Breathe in and hold your breath in for a moment.

Maintaining your gaze, slowly breathe out and lower your body into the extended position. Keep your lifted leg as far up and back as possible. Your left arm extends straight ahead. Your supporting leg remains straight. Stare at one spot for balance. Don't strain. Hold for a moment, then breathe in, come back to a standing position, and switch sides.

Alternate Triangle
(pictured, page 43)

Add this exercise between the Hip Rotation and the Side Triangle (pages 32–33). Maintain the Hip Rotation position with legs spread. Breathe in and stretch your arms out to the sides (as shown in Figure 4.11), then breathe out as you bend toward your right leg. Remember to keep your knees straight but not locked. Holding your breath out for a moment, grasp your right ankle firmly with both hands, bend your elbows, and pull gently, keeping your knees straight and tucking your chin into your chest (as shown in Figure 4.12). Breathe in as you return to the starting position. Repeat three times to each leg, alternating.

Lunge Series

Add this exercise between the Cobra V-Raise and the Baby Pose (pages 34–35). With your toes pointed inward, spread your legs as far apart as you comfortably can. Breathe in as you turn completely toward the left and bend your left leg, bringing your left elbow underneath your left knee and resting on both fists (Figure 4.31). Keep your right leg straight if you can; if that position is too strenuous, rest your knee on the floor. Bend your head toward the floor as you breathe out. Hold your breath out for a moment. Breathe in and release. Repeat on the opposite side.

Breathe in as you turn back to the left. Breathe out as you rest both elbows on the floor with your left elbow inside your left knee, lower your right knee to the floor, clasp your hands, and bend your head toward your hands (Figure 4.32). Hold your breath out for a moment.

Breathe in as you push yourself up, rest your left arm on your left thigh, and straighten your right arm and your right leg (Figure 4.33). Breathe out and hold your breath out for a moment.

Breathe in and release. With your legs in the same position, breathe out as you stretch both arms out to the sides, resting your chest on your left thigh (Figure 4.34). Hold your breath out for a moment.

Bring your left hand to the floor on the inside of your left leg. Breathe in and stretch your right arm straight up toward the ceiling (Figure 4.35). Look at your outstretched fingers and hold your breath in for a moment.

Breathe out, bring your arm down, swivel over to the right, and repeat the series facing right.

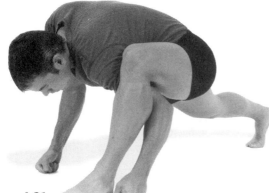

Figure 4.31

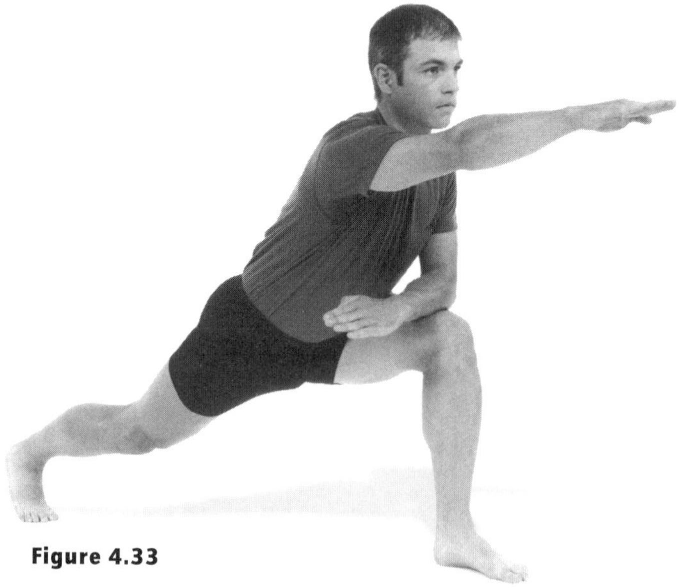

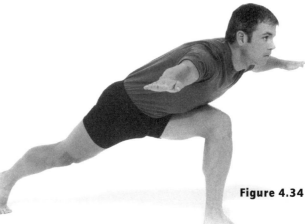

Figure 4.33

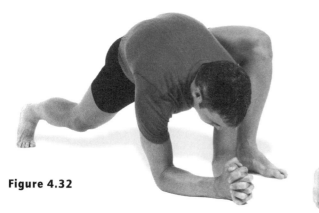

Figure 4.32

Figure 4.34

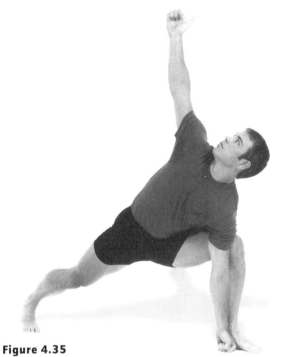

Figure 4.35

it across your left knee (Figure 4.37). Pull your left foot in close to your body.

Turn toward the right and bring your left arm over your right knee. With your left elbow, press your right knee back as far as it will comfortably go (Figure 4.38), then straighten your left arm and grasp the right big toe (Figure 4.39). If you can't reach your toe, grasp your ankle (Figure 4.40) or knee instead.

Spine Twist

Add the next two exercises between the Baby Pose and the Cobra Pose (pages 34–35). Sit up with both legs bent in front of you. Bend your left knee and lay it on the floor with your left foot under your right knee (Figure 4.36). Pick up your right foot and carry

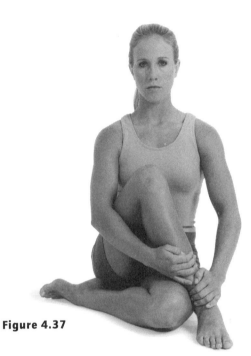

Figure 4.37

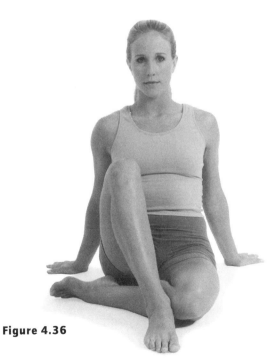

Figure 4.36

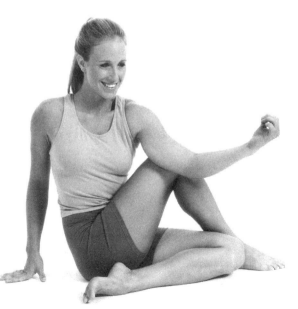

Figure 4.38

Bring your right hand close in to your body, fingers pointed in, and straighten your arm. Straighten your back, breathe in looking forward, then breathe out as you twist toward the right as far as you can without straining. Look at a spot on the wall just above eye level (Figure 4.41). Hold your breath out for a moment.

Release, and repeat on the opposite side.

Variation: for a less strenuous pose, keep the left leg outstretched (Figure 4.42).

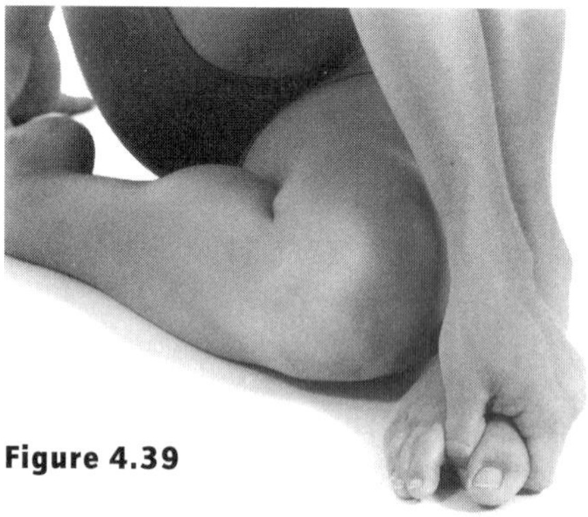

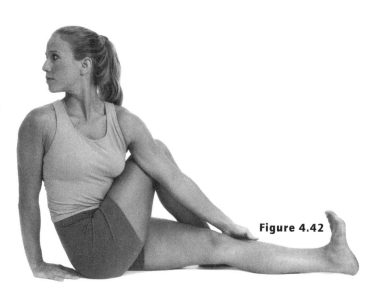

Figure 4.42

Figure 4.39

Figure 4.40

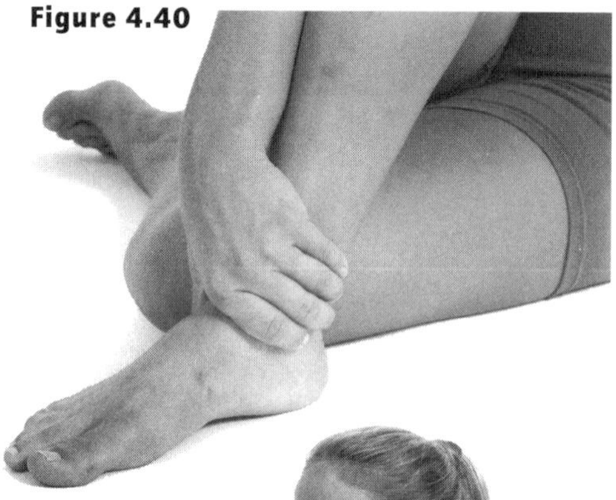

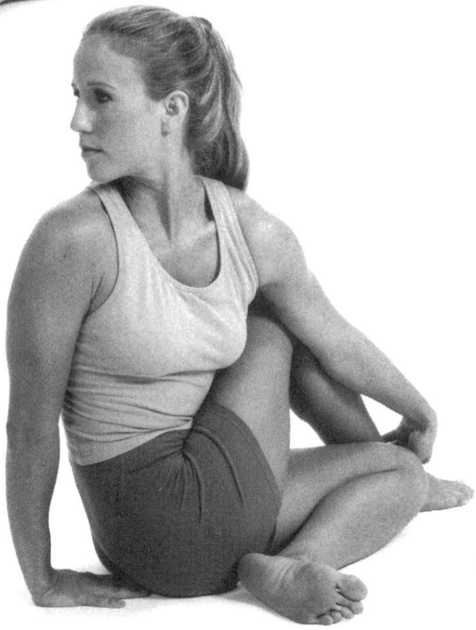

Diamond Pose

Sit with the soles of your feet together, knees relaxed outward, hands clasped around your toes (Figure 4.43). Breathe in and straighten your back, then breathe out and bend forward, bringing your head toward your feet and letting your elbows fall outside your knees (Figure 4.44). Tuck your chin into your throat, contract your rectal muscles, and hold your breath out for a moment. Breathe in and release. Repeat twice more.

To limber your hips and knees, grasp your ankles instead of your feet and, when you breathe out and bend forward, press down on your thighs with your elbows (Figure 4.45).

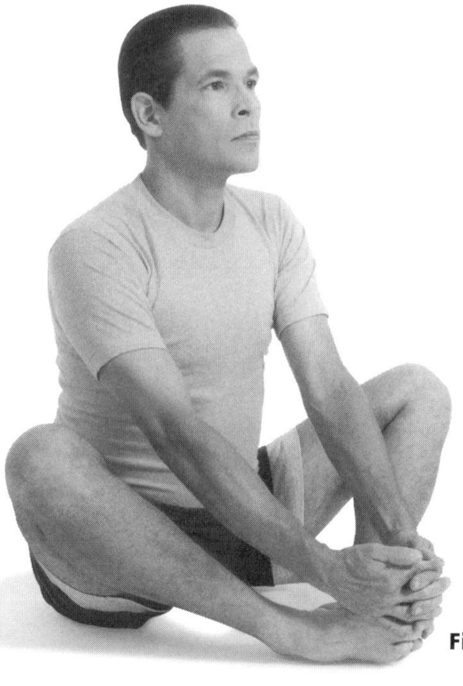

Figure 4.41

Figure 4.43

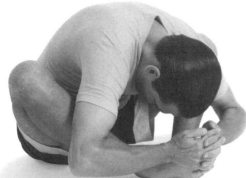

Figure 4.44

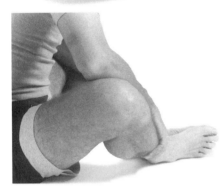

Figure 4.45

You don't have too much time to react as a catcher or a hitter. The thing about baseball that's tough is that the ball is not on the ground stationary, like golf, or like in basketball where the basket is stationary even though you are moving. The ball moves in many directions, at many different speeds, and that increases the ball break so it makes it very difficult. It almost becomes instincts that carry over more than just physical ability, so that you're able to read a pitch and then react to the pitch as a catcher or a player.

—Tommy Thompson, catching coach

Baseball/Softball

These sports require quick reaction time, a good sense of distance, and bursts of intense energy. Yoga exercise can stretch and strengthen the muscles of the back, legs, and abdomen; improve concentration and reaction time; and pull strength from the entire body to support the arm in use. Read the suggestions in Chapter 5 to help balance both sides of your body.

Running in spurts increases the risk of injury, especially if muscle strength is imbalanced. Pitchers are vulnerable to overuse injuries from repetitive throwing (mostly shoulder and elbow) and some-

times carpal tunnel problems. The best way to prevent these injuries is through general conditioning, stretching the shoulder and arm prior to the game, and daily practice of wrist and hand exercises.

Modify your core routine as follows:

Elbow Touch (pictured, page 57)
Add this exercise between the Shoulder Roll and the Elbow Twist (pages 28–29). Place your fingers on your shoulders, elbows out to the sides. Breathing normally, move your elbows toward each other in front, then squeeze them toward each other in back, keeping them at the same level. Repeat several times.

Full Bend Variation (pictured, page 57)
Add this exercise between the Neck Stretches and the Standing Sun Pose (pages 30–32). Stand with feet parallel. Clasp your hands behind your back. If you can, press your palms together. For an even greater stretch, lock your elbows so your shoulder blades are squeezed together. Breathe in and lift your arms in back as far as you can without straining. Breathe out and bend forward, tucking your chin and keeping your arms in position. Hold your breath out for a moment. Breathe in and straighten. Repeat the exercise twice more.

Bow Variation
Add this exercise between the Cat Breath and the Cobra V-Raise (page 34). Start on your hands and knees. Reach back with your left hand and grasp your right foot. Stare at one spot on the wall or floor for balance as you breathe in and lift your foot up

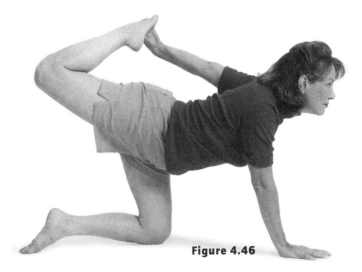

Figure 4.46

TARGET ATHLETES IMPROVE MUSCLE CONTROL

Does your sport demand the ultimate in precision? B-complex vitamin supplementation has significantly benefited fine-motor control and also reduced muscle tremor, resulting in improved performance of precision sports. Always keep B-complex vitamins in balance. Keep in mind that niacinamide is superior to niacin and that high levels of vitamin B_6 (more than 10 mg per day) may actually reduce endurance performance. Use the following as a daily guide:

Vitamin B_1 (thiamin) 100–1,000 mg
Vitamin B_2 (riboflavin) 10–100 mg
Vitamin B_3 (niacinamide) 22 mg

Pantothenate (pantothenic acid) 50–2,000 mg
Vitamin B_6 (pyridoxine) 2–10 mg
Vitamin B_{12} (cyanocobalamin) 2–100 mcg
Folate (folic acid) 400–800 mcg

Thiamine and Pantothenate have shown some performance-enhancing effects for a wide range of sports. The other B vitamins are included at safe levels to prevent possible imbalances. At 10 mg. daily, vitamin B_6 may have a positive impact on "burst" activity such as weight lifting and football line play.

and away from your body as far as possible (Figure 4.46). Hold your breath in for a moment. Breathe out, release slowly, and switch sides. Repeat three times on each side.

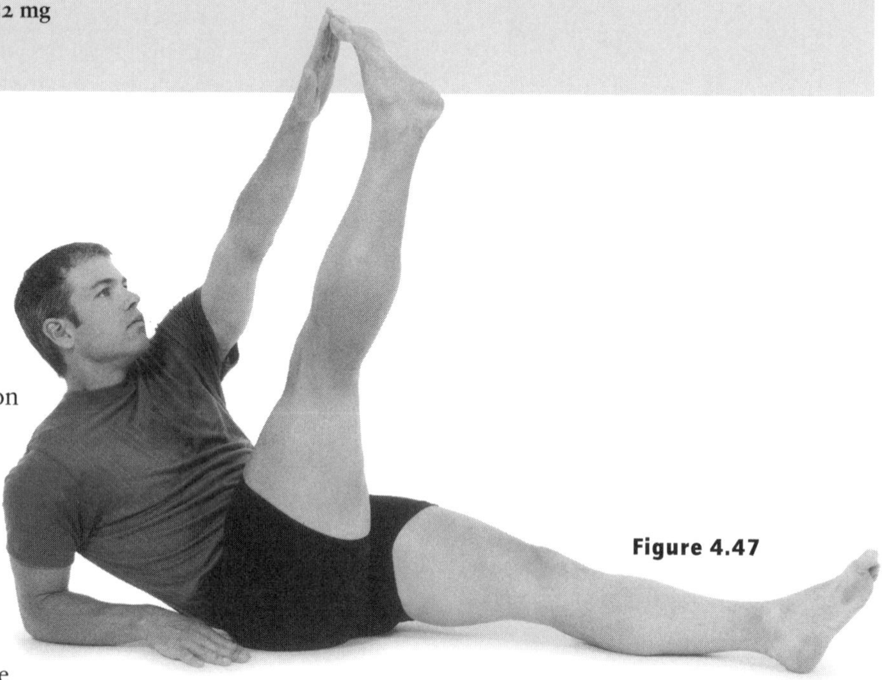

Boat Pose (pictured, page 75)

Add this exercise between the Baby Pose and the Cobra Pose (pages 34–35). Lying on your stomach, stretch your arms on the floor over your head and place your forehead on the floor. Breathe out. Breathe in as you lift your arms, legs, and head, looking up through your forehead. Hold your breath in for a moment. Breathe out and release, bringing your arms and forehead back to the floor. Repeat twice more.

Figure 4.47

Alternate Big Sit-Up

Add the next two exercises between the Cobra Pose and the Knee Squeeze (pages 35–36). Lie on your back with your arms at your sides. Bring your left arm over your head on the floor and breathe out.

Breathe in as you lift your left arm and right leg (opposites) and touch your toes, supporting yourself on your right elbow (Figure 4.47). Hold your breath in for a moment. Breathe out and lower. Repeat three times on each side.

Easy Bridge and Wheel

Lying on your back, bend your knees and separate your legs and feet several inches; place your arms at your sides, palms down (Figure 4.48). Breathe in, then breathe out as you lift your hips, arching your

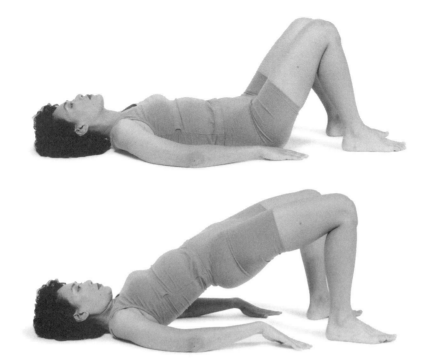

Figure 4.48

Figure 4.49

back and tucking your chin into your chest (Figure 4.49). Hold your breath out for a moment. Repeat twice more.

Variation: if you are very limber, you can grasp your ankles with both hands.

If you are strong enough, try the Wheel: place your hands next to your head, fingers pointing toward your feet (Figure 4.50). Breathe in and push up so you are resting on your head (Figure 4.51). If you can, continue pushing up into the full position (Figure 4.52). Hold your breath in for a moment.

Breathe out and lower your body to the floor, straighten your legs, bring your arms down to your sides, and rest.

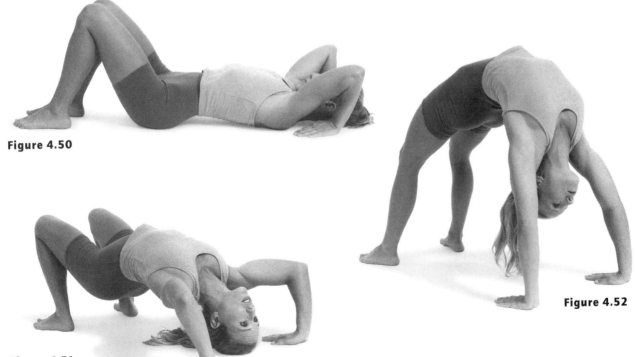

Figure 4.50

Figure 4.51

Figure 4.52

Hand Limbering Exercises

Add this exercise after the Knee Squeeze (page 36).
Repeat each of the following movements several
times. Spread your fingers wide apart (Figure 4.53),
then make fists (Figure 4.54). Press the fingers of one
hand back using the opposite hand (Figure 4.55).
Repeat on the opposite side. Make a "steeple"
with your fingers and press the fingers together
(Figure 4.56).

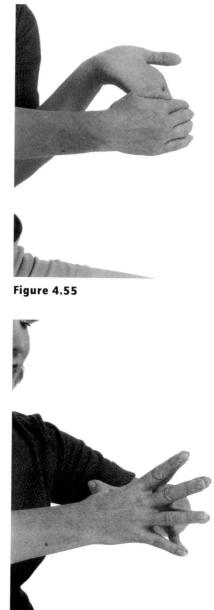

Figure 4.55

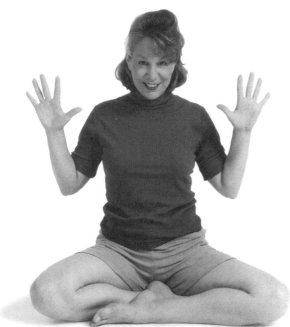

Figure 4.53

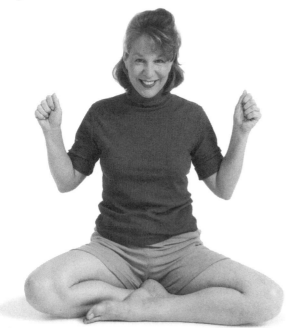

Figure 4.54

Figure 4.56

Volleyball

This game involves bursts of quick movement in
many directions, using many of the same muscle
movements as tennis. Yoga exercises will strengthen
and stretch the leg muscles, maintain a strong back,
and balance both sides of the body. Yoga breathing
exercises can improve stamina and increase feelings
of fluid team participation.

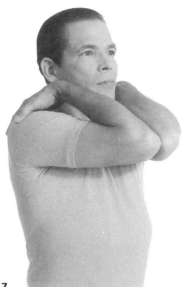

Figure 4.57

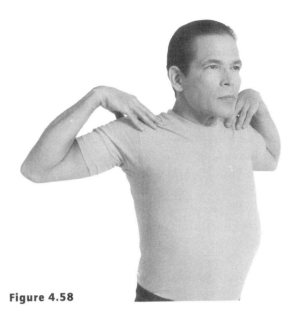

Figure 4.58

Volleyball players often experience sore shoulders from overhead play, back strain, and jumper's knee from constant bending. The best way to prevent these injuries is through general conditioning, stretching and strengthening of the legs, back, and shoulders.

Modify your core routine as follows:

Elbow Touch

Add this exercise between the Shoulder Roll and the Elbow Twist (pages 28–29). Place your fingers on your shoulders, elbows out to the sides. Breathing normally, move your elbows toward each other in front (Figure 4.57), then squeeze them toward each other in back (Figure 4.58), keeping them at the same level. Repeat several times.

Full Bend Variation

Add this exercise between the Neck Stretches and the Standing Sun Pose (pages 30–32). Stand with feet parallel. Clasp your hands behind your back. If you can, press your palms together. For an even greater stretch, lock your elbows so your shoulder blades are squeezed together. Breathe in and lift your arms in back as far as you can without straining

Figure 4.59

(Figure 4.59). Breathe out and bend forward, tucking your chin and keeping your arms in position (Figure 4.60). Hold your breath out for a moment. Breathe in and straighten. Repeat the exercise twice more.

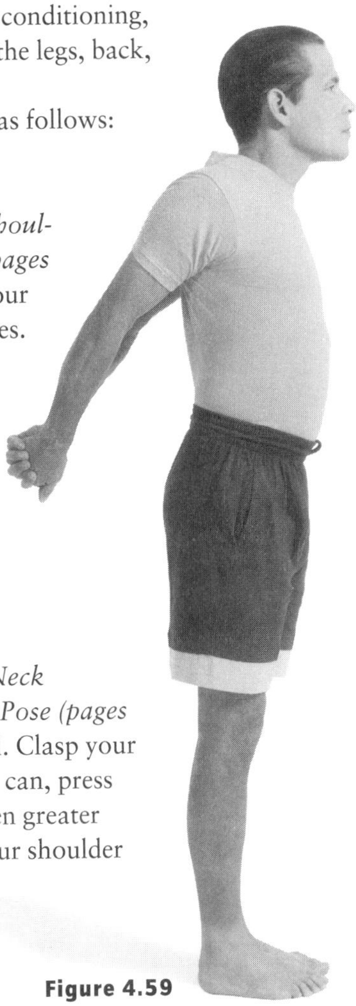

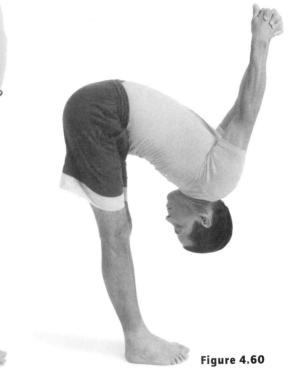

Figure 4.60

T Pose (pictured, page 48)

Add the next two exercises between the Twisting Triangle and the Cat Breath (pages 33–34). When you are first learning this position, stand three to four feet from a chair or other support. Lean forward and hold on to the support with both hands. Lift your left leg in back as high as you can, ideally, parallel to the floor. Alternatively, brace yourself with both hands on the knee of your supporting leg. Keep your right (supporting) leg straight. Your torso and left leg should be in a straight line parallel to the floor. Keep your neck straight, breathe naturally, and look at a spot on the floor.

When you feel steady, release your grip on the support and place your palms together, pushing your arms out parallel to the floor. Relax your breath. Look forward at your hands. Lower your leg and return to a standing position. Rest until your breath returns to normal. Repeat on the opposite side.

Knee Bends

From the T Pose position, breathing naturally, keep your torso and lifted leg straight and parallel to the floor and, clasping your hands behind your back, gently bend your right knee and straighten (Figure 4.61). Try to do this without letting your shoulders and head bend toward the floor while your knee is bent. Keep breathing naturally. Stand up and rest. Repeat up to three times. Repeat on the opposite side.

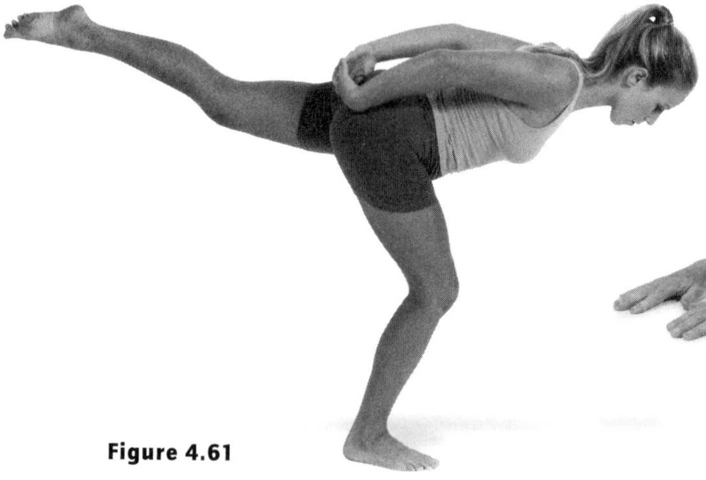

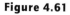

Figure 4.61

Spine Twist (pictured, pages 51–52)

Add the next two exercises between the Baby Pose and the Cobra Pose (pages 34–35). Sit up with both legs bent in front of you. Bend your left knee and lay it on the floor with your left foot under your right knee. Pick up your right foot and carry it across your left knee. Pull your left foot in close to your body.

Turn toward the right and bring your left arm over your right knee. With your left elbow, press your right knee back as far as it will comfortably go, then straighten your left arm and grasp the right big toe. If you can't reach your toe, grasp your ankle or knee instead.

Bring your right hand close in to your body, fingers pointed in, and straighten your arm. Straighten your back, breathe in looking forward, then breathe out as you twist toward the right as far as you can without straining. Look at a spot on the wall just above eye level. Hold your breath out for a moment.

Release, and repeat on the opposite side.

Variation: for a less strenuous pose, keep the left leg outstretched.

Back Strengthener Series

Stretch your arms on the floor over your head and place your forehead on the floor (Figure 4.62). Breathe out. Breathe in as you lift your arms, legs, and head, looking up through your forehead (Figure 4.63; this exercise is also called the Boat Pose). Hold your breath in for a moment.

Breathe out and release, bringing both arms straight out to the sides, palms down, and forehead to the floor (Figure 4.64). Rest a moment, then breathe in as you lift your arms, legs, and head, looking up through your forehead (Figure 4.65). Hold your breath in for a moment.

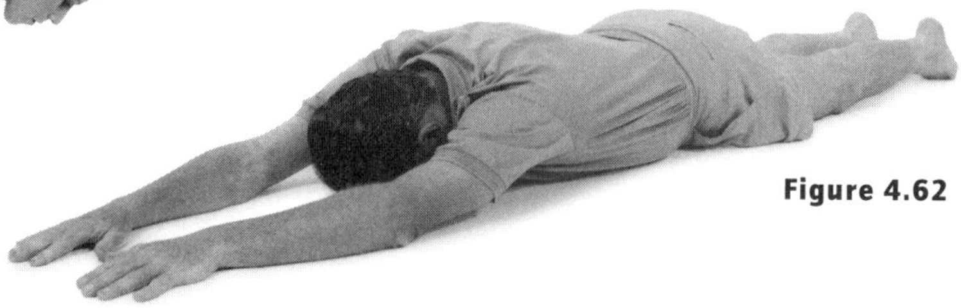

Figure 4.62

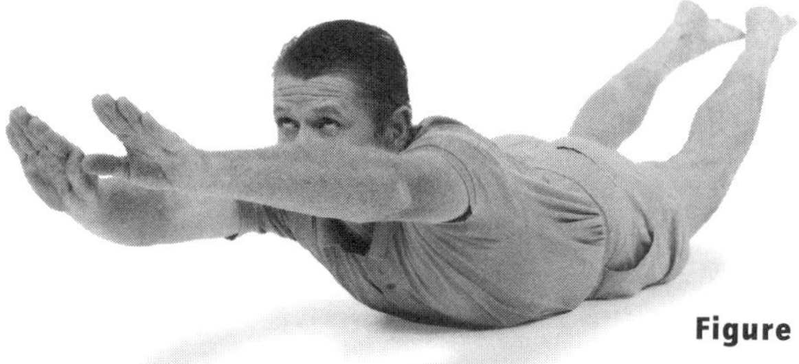

Figure 4.63

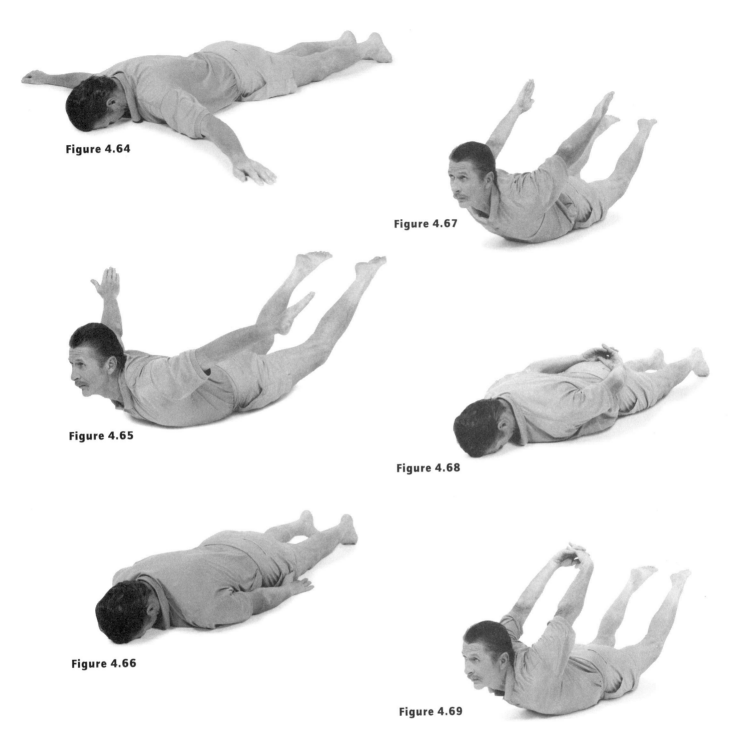

Figure 4.64

Figure 4.67

Figure 4.65

Figure 4.68

Figure 4.66

Figure 4.69

Breathe out and release, bringing your arms down to your sides (Figure 4.66). Rest a moment, then breathe in as you lift your arms, legs, and head, looking up through your forehead (Figure 4.67). Hold your breath in for a moment.

Breathe out and release, bringing your arms behind your back with your fingers clasped (Figure 4.68). Rest a moment, then breathe in as you lift your arms, legs, and head, pressing your palms together and straightening your arms as much as possible so your shoulder blades are squeezed together and your arms stretch away from your body (Figure 4.69). Look up through your forehead. Hold your breath in for a moment.

Breathe out and release, bending your knees and grasping your feet with both hands (Figure 4.70). Rest a moment with your forehead to the floor, then breathe in as you lift, pulling up on your feet so you balance on your stomach (Figure 4.71; this position is also called the Bow Pose.) Look up through your forehead. Hold your breath in for a moment. Breathe out and release. Rest on your stomach.

Humming Breath

Add this exercise after the Knee Squeeze (page 36). Sit up in a comfortable position, either cross-legged or sitting on your feet, or sit on the edge of a chair with your hands on your knees. Breathe in completely just as you would in the Complete Breath, described on page 20. Now breathe out with an audible *hummmm* sound, making the tone steady and loud until your breath is gone—just like the sound of a bumblebee. Let the sound vibrate in your throat, and keep pushing with your belly muscles so that the sound doesn't trail off at the end. Try to keep the sound steady. Repeat several times.

Basketball

Basketball is discussed in Chapter 6, "Endurance Sports."

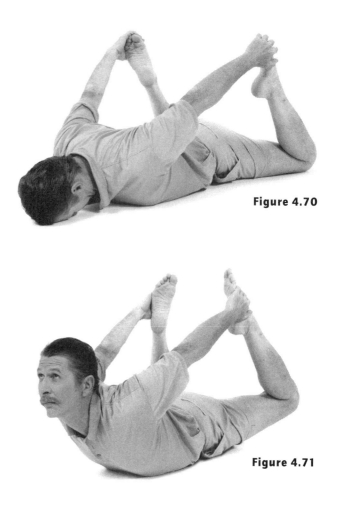

Figure 4.70

Figure 4.71

5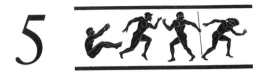

SPORTS USING ONE SIDE OF THE BODY

Tennis and Other Racquet Sports, Field Hockey, Ice Hockey, Throwing Events, Bowling, and Golf

When you're in peak performance it feels like everything else is in slow motion. You're going at a different speed than the events around you.

—ARTIE GUERIN

I would always use visualization before, during, and after a game to visualize a serve, foul shot, or softball swing. I would often not only visualize my movements and actions but also those of my teammates and what I needed from them to make the shot or block a success.

—ALICE KENNEDY

It is easy to see that if you direct extreme effort to one side of your body repeatedly, the opposite side of the body will not be as strong. This means that constant training in balance of the two sides is a necessity for success in the game. In the final effort, you will not be able to engage your target effectively without using your entire body. This chapter gives you a concentration technique that mentally employs your whole body and makes your game much more effective.

If you are a tennis player, or a practitioner of other racquet sports, you will find that your serves and other shots can be more accurate and powerful if you use the art of concentration to engage your whole body in each stroke. Golfers and hockey players have an edge in that both hands are used for play, and so greater balance is available for them to work with. Even so, the concentration training outlined in this chapter will increase the power of play for these athletes as well. Concentration training is easy to do and can become a pleasant addition to your everyday practice. I recommend that you use it before your practice session as part of your warmup routine.

Concentration Technique

Sit on the floor with your back against a wall, or sit in a straight-back chair. It is important to keep your spine straight and your head in line with your spine. For best results, practice when you are alone, or at least in a quiet, undisturbed place. Close your eyes and take a few deep breaths. Then let yourself relax and let your breathing relax into its regular rhythm.

As you begin to relax, slowly become aware of your breathing and visualize the breath going to both sides of your body with your mental direction. Begin with your nondominant side: start with a particular spot on your head and begin at the same spot each time you practice the exercise. Picture in fantasy the breath moving through all your nerves, bones, and muscles on that side. Slowly, mentally move the breath force all the way down the side of your body into your leg and foot.

Then, while concentrated at that point, simply stop and do nothing. Simply concentrate on the breath reaching your foot. Don't move your mind to anything or anywhere else, and don't talk to yourself. Hold that point for a minute or two, then move

Basketball is the biggest sport in which I use my visualization techniques. I visualize my foul shots before every game, and even at night before I go to bed, basically whenever I can. I picture myself in the game, standing at the foul line with the ball. I picture myself doing my foul shot routine, and then I picture myself putting the ball in the net.

—Eve Kennedy, basketball and other team-sports player

your visual concentration to your other foot. Slowly bring your breath back up through the opposite side of your body to your starting point in your head. You will soon feel the improved balance of the body in your daily sport activity.

Breath is the source of strength, and although the physical body is the machinery that operates with that strength, the *source* of breath is actually the emotional/spiritual/power body. Concentration training with the technique outlined above will bring about a melded effort of breath, using the two bodies that have now formed a powerful whole. This will give full strength to your athletic effort. Use this technique daily to encourage a natural support and expression of strength using the whole body in your game and to create the perfect balance that is needed for outstanding sports experience.

Concentration training using your breath will give you results quickly. For an even greater effect, try the following additional fantasy technique:

Fantasy Technique

After performing the breath concentration exercise starting on the nondominant side of your body, and completing through the dominant side, mentally envision the breath entering all parts of your body—both sides—and then envision your entire body filled with breath strength. Then go one step further. Keeping your eyes closed, and sitting very still with your back straight, picture yourself in the game as you wish yourself to be. Practice a difficult serve, get yourself out of a tricky sand trap, or see yourself performing the lightning-quick reactions needed for brilliant play in your sport. Form a clear picture of yourself succeeding.

Once you are able to realize a clear picture of yourself doing what you want to do, the way you want to do it, then purposefully enjoy that moment in your whole body. Stop all thought, all fantasy, and all talking to yourself. Be completely silent in your physical and emotional body for a moment or two. Allow the fantasy of complete success to flood your whole body and mind. Your breath will change slightly at this moment. Then slowly resume a natural breath pattern, open your eyes, and slowly prepare to start toward your game. You will find that you feel no nervousness about your approach, and you will become aware of a strong, quiet, and enjoyable confidence from within. You will have made a bridge to your inner emotional body, which will allow you now to feel the full support of both your physical and emotional natures. This will give you complete strength for the game.

Eventually, as you make this bridge of connection with your inner self, the full force of breath will automatically occupy both sides of your body equally, giving you great strength and balance.

Another way to balance both sides of your body is to sometimes practice playing your sport using your nondominant side. Although it will feel awkward at first, balancing the strength of your body in this way will improve your performance. Using your nondominant side for at least 5 to 10 minutes during training will make your performance much stronger and more accurate when you return to training with your dominant side.

> *Trying to play with my nondominant hand definitely helped me understand the pitfalls that people have. When I played left-handed, which is my dominant side, it was so effortless how I timed the ball. But when I tried to do it right-handed, knowing that my backhand shot is harder right-handed, my body flinched. It went into a spastic sort of motion which I immediately recognized in all my students. They had trouble not only with just one shot but a lot of them with everything. So it helped me understand and appreciate the difficulties of learning.*
>
> —Artie Guerin

Training on your nondominant side will, of course, not always result in the expert functioning of your primary side, but it will show you several interesting features. First, it takes more concentration to achieve your goal. This training gives strong support to your ability to perform because you learn how to give extreme concentrated effort to all the parts of your body, not just one side; and you can achieve your goal with less effort. Concentration then will become natural; you won't have to force it. The power of concentration will be much more easily available to you at all times.

Second, by supplying extra attention and training to the nondominant side of your body, your body strength becomes redistributed, rather than one-sided. This provides a solid block of support to your final effort. You achieve your goal with your whole body, not with one arm or one side of your body. This results in a much stronger performance.

A third helpful result of whole-body training is that it quickens awareness. Change and flexibility are the natural products of awareness, and these qualities are crucial for expert performance.

The best result of all this is that when you return to your natural dominant side, it will be much easier to achieve your mark. It is almost as if the side of your body that you use naturally shows the other side how to do it. Gradually your nondominant side will begin to show its strength and accuracy and will become totally supportive in your athletic efforts.

The Sport Routines

The exercises in the following routines focus on techniques that will help athletes balance both sides of their body and stay strong and limber. For best results, always include a few minutes of breathing and meditation in your daily Yogic routine.

Tennis/Racquetball

Racquet sports require great intuitive coordination, timing, strength, and agility, as the player must react and move quickly in all directions over the course of a game. Yoga exercises can help balance both sides of the body; strengthen legs, knees, and back; and provide overall training in flexibility. Meditation and breathing will bring on intuitive force.

TIPS FOR DEALING WITH TENNIS ELBOW

The majority of people who play tennis at one time or another experience some form of elbow pain, and although some serious cases may require drastic measures such as surgery, there are some less invasive ways to cure the problem.

Tennis elbow is an inflammation of the tendons that attach the forearm muscle to the bony knob on the outside of the elbow. Other activities such as gardening, playing a musical instrument, carpentry, writing, and using a computer keyboard can also cause this problem. If you are a tennis player, have a professional look closely at your equipment and your technique—sometimes the problem is easy to diagnose and correct.

To minimize further damage to the forearm muscles:

1. Stretch out and warm up your arms and shoulders before play with exercises such as Shoulder Rolls (p. 28), Arm Circles (p. 30), and Hand-Limbering Exercises (p. 56). A properly fitted elbow sleeve may help. Salves such as Ben-Gay or Tiger Balm will warm up the area, promoting blood circulation.
2. Ice down your elbow immediately after play to limit inflammation. If ice is not readily available, just use an ice-cold beverage can.
3. Rest between days of play. Remember, the pain and discomfort are caused by inflammation, so let it subside before you use your elbow again.

There is no one cure for tennis elbow; if your inflammation is mild, you may be able to use some natural therapies such as vitamin C, herbs, or calcium to reduce the inflammation. Acupuncture, acupressure, various types of massage, and other nonsurgical treatments may also help. On a short-term, occasional basis, aspirin, ibuprofen, or stronger drugs can be effective in reducing inflammation. However, even over-the-counter drugs should be used with a doctor's supervision, and they only mask the pain; they do not cure the problem.

Once the inflammation has receded, you can start a resistance exercise program followed by stretching exercises for the forearm muscles to help avoid recurrence.

[This section was abridged from a longer article with permission of the author, Artie Guerin. For information on obtaining the complete article, see Resources.]

Quick movements in different directions make tennis and racquetball players prone to knee and foot injuries; players may also experience repetitive motion problems and injuries to the shoulder and elbow. The best way to prevent these injuries is to strengthen the back and legs and follow an all-around flexibility and strength routine. See the sidebar "Tips for Dealing with Tennis Elbow" above, for information on treating this common injury among players of racquet sports.

Modify your core routine as follows:

Lunge Series (pictured, pages 70–71)
Add this exercise between the Twisting Triangle and the Cat Breath (pages 33–34). With your toes pointed inward, spread your legs as far apart as you comfortably can. Breathe in as you turn completely toward the left and bend your left leg, bringing your left elbow underneath your left knee and resting on both fists. Keep your right leg straight if you can; if that position is too strenuous, rest your knee on the floor. Bend your head toward the floor as you breathe out. Hold your breath out for a moment. Breathe in and release. Repeat on the opposite side.

Breathe in as you turn back to the left. Breathe out as you rest both elbows on the floor with your left elbow inside your left knee, lower your right knee to the floor, clasp your hands, and bend your head toward your hands. Hold your breath out for a moment.

Breathe in as you push yourself up, rest your left arm on your left thigh, and straighten your right arm and your right leg. Breathe out and hold your breath out for a moment.

Breathe in and release. With your legs in the same position, breathe out as you stretch both arms out to the sides, resting your chest on your left thigh. Hold your breath out for a moment.

Bring your left hand to the floor on the inside of your left leg. Breathe in and stretch your right arm straight up toward the ceiling. Look at your out-stretched fingers and hold your breath in for a moment.

Breathe out, bring your arm down, swivel over to the right, and repeat the series facing right.

Lion Pose

Add the next four exercises between the Baby Pose and the Cobra Pose (pages 34–35). Sit on your feet, or cross-legged. Spread your fingers apart like a lion's paws and grip your knees. Lean forward slightly and take a deep breath through your nose. Open your eyes wide, raise your eyebrows, stick out your tongue, and roar fiercely (Figure 5.1). Visualize and try to look like a roaring lion.

Spine Twist

Sit up with both legs bent in front of you. Bend your left knee and lay it on the floor with your left foot under your right knee (Figure 5.2). Pick up your right foot and carry it across your left knee (Figure 5.3). Pull your left foot in close to your body.

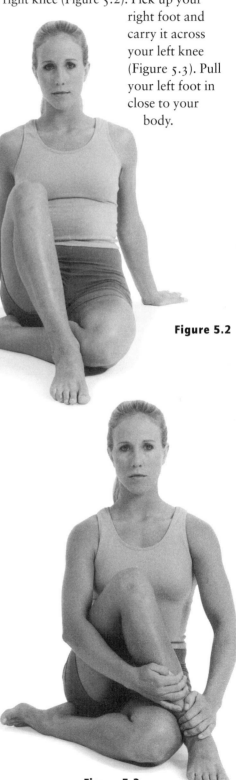

Figure 5.2

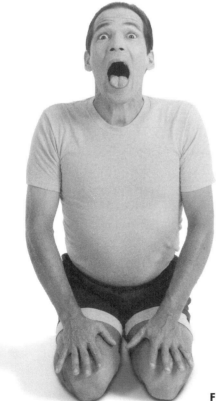

Figure 5.1

Figure 5.3

Turn toward the right and bring your left arm over your right knee. With your left elbow, press your right knee back as far as it will comfortably go (Figure 5.4), then straighten your left arm and grasp the right big toe (Figure 5.5). If you can't reach your toe, grasp your ankle (Figure 5.6) or knee instead.

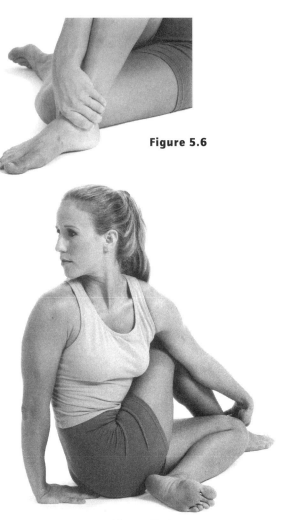

Figure 5.6

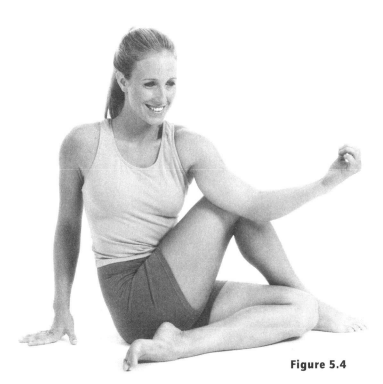

Figure 5.4

Figure 5.7

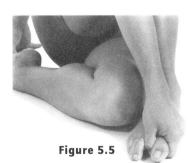

Figure 5.5

on the wall just above eye level (Figure 5.7). Hold your breath out for a moment. Release, and repeat on the opposite side.

Variation: for a less strenuous pose, keep the left leg outstretched (Figure 5.8).

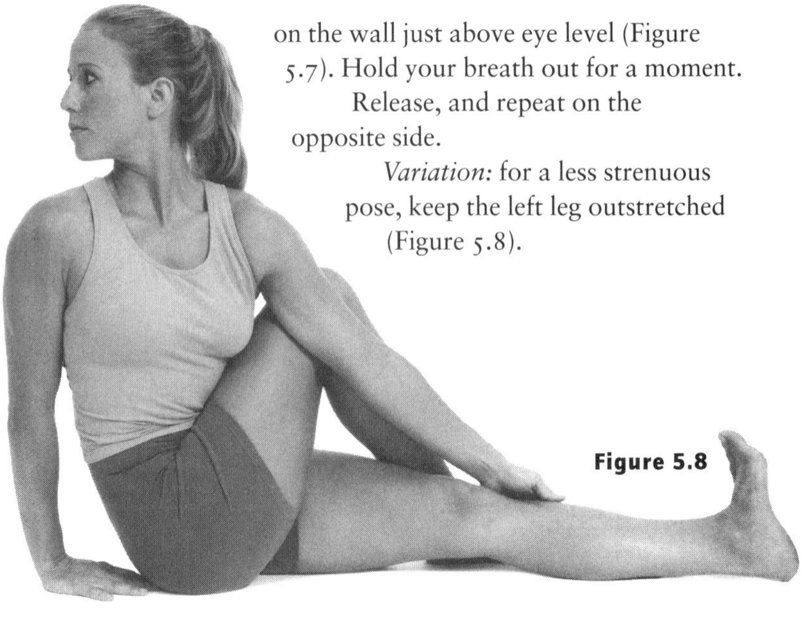

Bring your right hand close in to your body, fingers pointed in, and straighten your arm. Straighten your back, breathe in looking forward, then breath out as you twist toward the right as far as you can without straining. Look at a spot

Figure 5.8

Seated Sun Pose
(pictured, pages 71–72)

Bring both legs straight out in front of you and flex your toes. Sit straight, breathe out with your arms at your sides, then breathe in as you raise your arms in a wide circle to the sides and overhead. Press your palms together, look up, visualize the sun, and stretch from the rib cage. Hold your breath in for a moment.

Breathe out as you bend forward, tucking your chin toward your chest. Grasp your ankles, bend your elbows, and pull your torso toward your legs (remember to pull by bending your arms, not by pushing with your lower back). Hold your breath out for a moment.

If you are limber enough to reach your feet (and still bend your elbows), grasp your big toes as shown on page 72.

Release and breathe in, bringing your arms to the sides and over your head again. Stretch and look up as before. Breathe out and bring your arms back down to your sides. Repeat three times.

Bow Pose

Lie on your stomach with your forehead to the floor. Bend your knees and grasp your ankles or feet with your hands (Figure 5.9; you may have to separate your legs slightly to reach). Breathe in as you lift and look up, pulling up on your feet so you balance on your stomach. Look up through your forehead (Figure 5.10). Visualize yourself as a bow. Hold

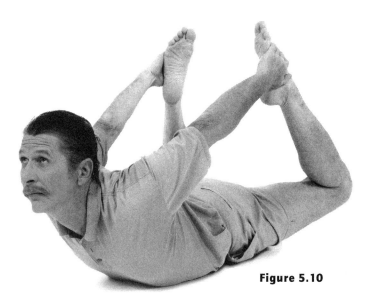

Figure 5.10

your breath in for a moment. Breathe out and release. Repeat twice more.

Alternate Big Sit-Up
(pictured, page 105)

Add the next two exercises after the Knee Squeeze (page 36). Lie on your back with your arms at your sides. Bring your left arm over your head on the floor and breathe out. Breathe in as you lift your left arm and right leg (opposites) and touch your toes, supporting yourself on your right elbow. Hold your breath in for a moment. Breathe out and lower. Repeat three times on each side.

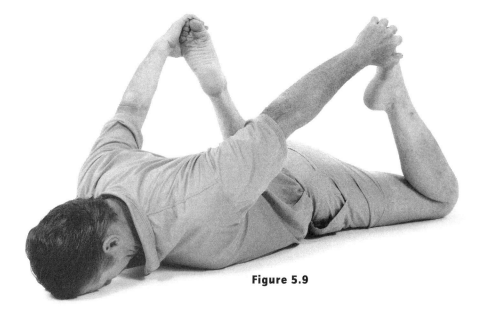

Figure 5.9

Hand-Limbering Exercises

Repeat each of the following movements several times. Spread your fingers wide apart (Figure 5.11), then make fists (Figure 5.12). Press the fingers of one

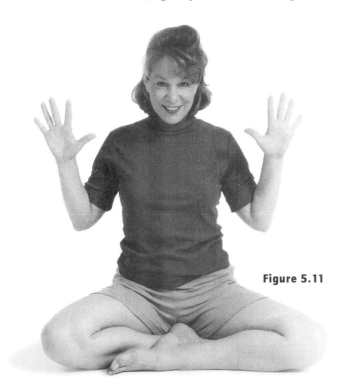

Figure 5.11

Tennis was much more difficult for me emotionally because there's so much time in between the movement phases that there's time to get your ego involved and to lose that focus of the moment. So I had to learn tricks in tennis to teach me to not lose my focus. What worked for me—because I was very emotional and easily distracted—was when I would put myself into a sort of meditative state before I played. I would lie down and gradually relax my body, my toes up to my head. And then I'd visualize all the common things that I had done wrong in the past. And then I would visualize the successful demeanor on my part and performance. That would sort of take root in my head. And then I would try to stay totally within myself. So when I'd go to play a game, I wouldn't get involved with the other player, because that would take me out of that state.

—Artie Guerin

hand back using the opposite hand (Figure 5.13). Repeat on the opposite side. Make a "steeple" with your fingers and press the fingers together (Figure 5.14).

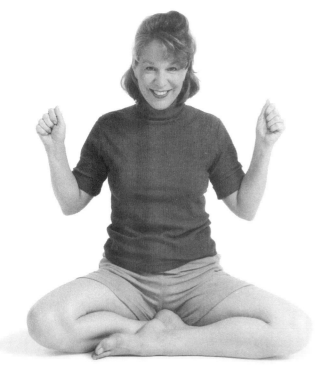

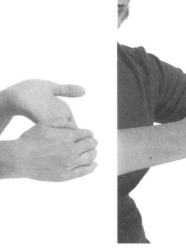

Figure 5.12   Figure 5.13   Figure 5.14

Field Hockey/Ice Hockey

Ice hockey is a fast, rough game that requires speed, strength, and quick reactions. Field hockey, played on grass, requires stamina and endurance. For athletes who play either type of hockey, Yoga can help balance both sides of the body; improve concentration, stamina, reaction time, and awareness; and provide overall strength and flexibility training.

Ice hockey injuries result mainly from contact with other players or equipment; in addition, the constant bent-over position can create lower back pain. Field hockey injuries stem mainly from muscle strains and pulls. The best way to prevent these injuries is through an all-around routine promoting flexibility and strength, emphasizing the knees, ankles, and back.

Modify your core routine as follows:

Complete Breath with Arm Circles

Add this exercise before the Shoulder Roll (pages 28–29). Sit in a comfortable position as described in Chapter 2, page 20. Begin the Complete Breath exercise, but add this component: as you breathe in, raise your arms in circles to the sides and over your head. At the top, hold your breath in for just a moment as you stretch up with your fists (Figure 5.15). Then breathe out as you lower your arms in a circle back to the floor. Repeat three to five times.

Leg Raises

Add this exercise between the Neck Stretches and the Standing Sun Pose (pages 30–32). Stand

Figure 5.16

straight with both hands on your hips. (If you feel unsteady, you can hold on to a chair with your right hand.) Breathe out completely. Breathe in as you lift your right leg straight up in front as high as possible without bending your knee or straining (Figure 5.16). Hold the position and your breath for a moment. Breathe out and lower your leg. Breathe in and lift your right leg straight out to the side as far as possible without straining (Figure 5.17).

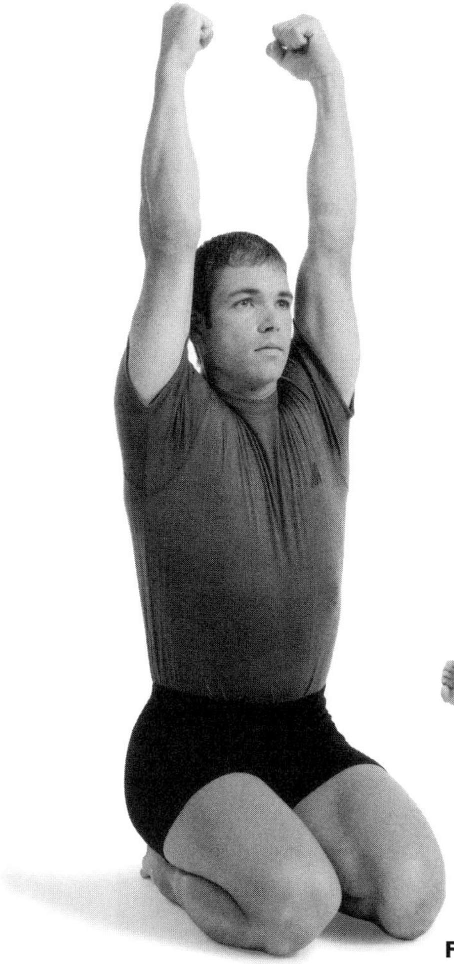

Figure 5.15

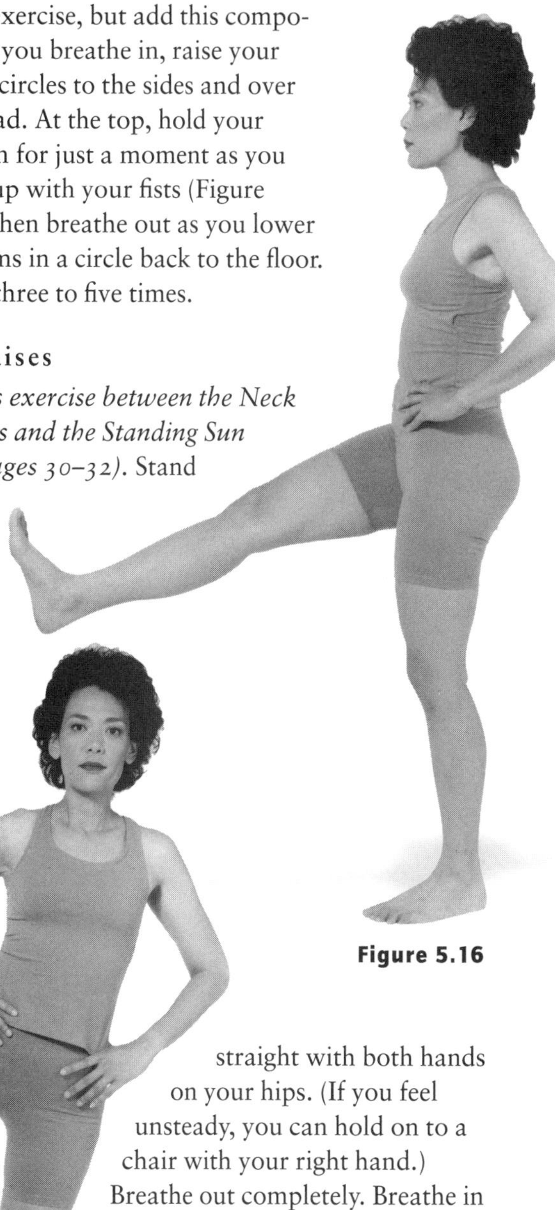

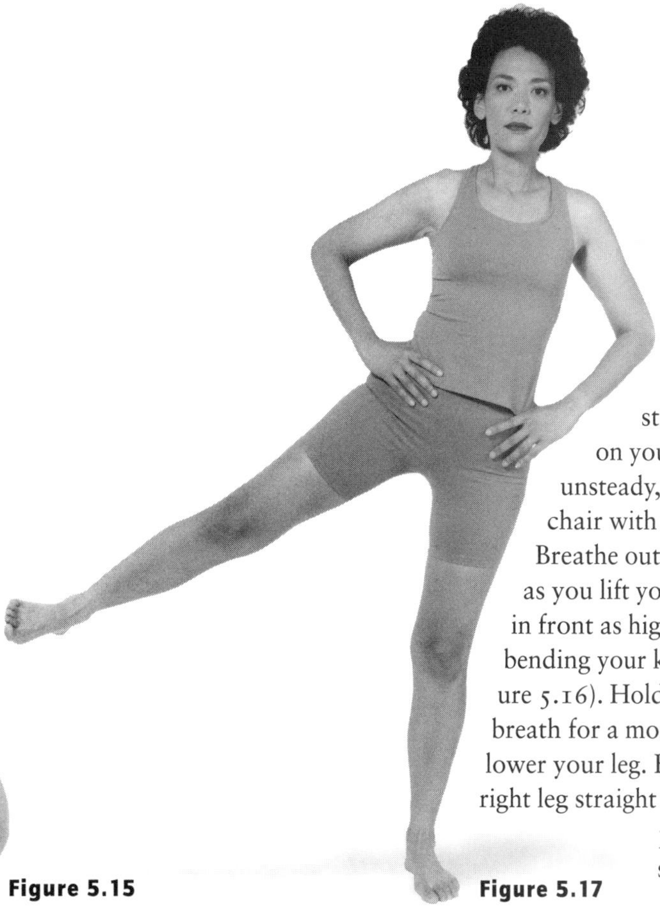

Figure 5.17

Hold the position and your breath for a moment. Breathe out and lower your leg. Breathe in and lift your right leg straight out in back as far as possible without bending your knee (Figure 5.18). Hold the position and your breath for a moment. Breathe out and lower your leg. Repeat with your left leg.

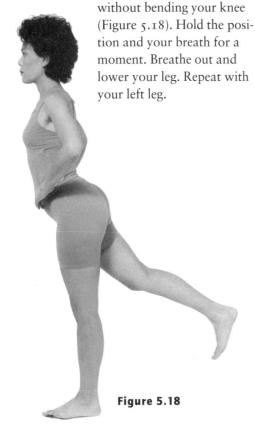

Figure 5.18

Lunge Series

Add this exercise between the Twisting Triangle and the Cat Breath (pages 33–34). With your toes pointed inward, spread your legs as far apart as you comfortably can. Breathe in as you turn completely toward the left and bend your left leg, bringing your left elbow underneath your left knee and resting on both fists (Figure 5.19). Keep your right leg straight if you can; if that position is too strenuous, rest your knee on the floor. Bend your head toward the floor as you breathe out.

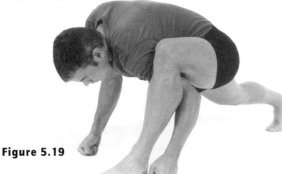

Figure 5.19

Hold your breath out for a moment. Breathe in and release. Repeat on the opposite side.

Breathe in as you turn back to the left. Breathe out as you rest both elbows on the floor with your left elbow inside your left knee, lower your right knee to the floor, clasp your hands, and bend your head toward your hands (Figure 5.20). Hold your breath out for a moment.

Breathe in as you push yourself up, rest your left arm on your left thigh, and straighten your right arm and your right leg (Figure 5.21). Breathe out and hold your breath out for a moment.

Breathe in and release. With your legs in the same position, breathe out as you stretch both arms out to the sides, resting your chest on your left thigh (Figure 5.22).

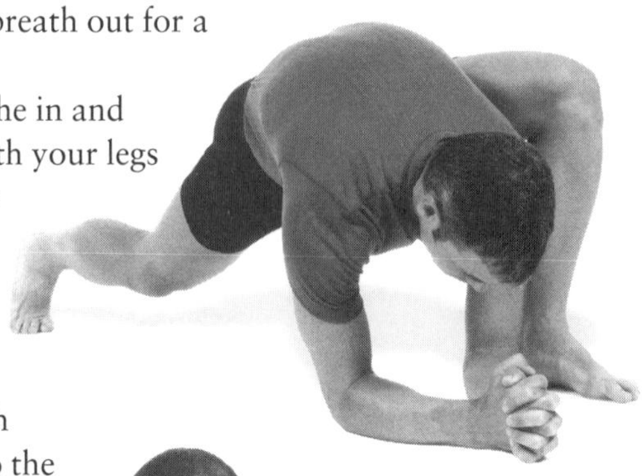

Figure 5.20

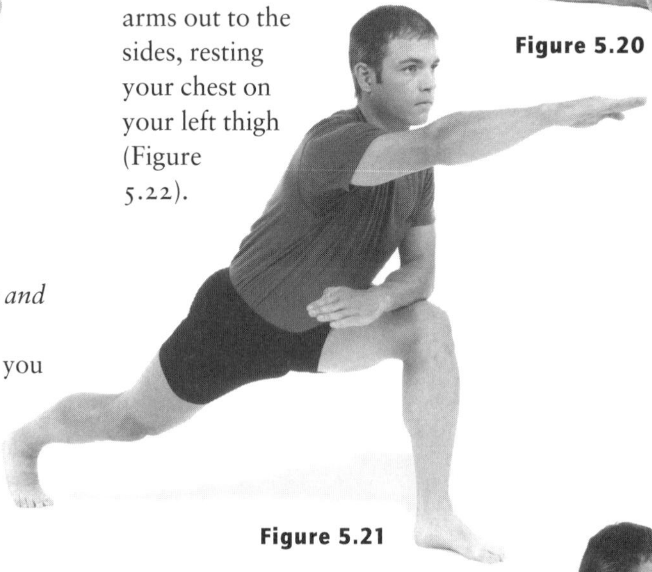

Figure 5.21

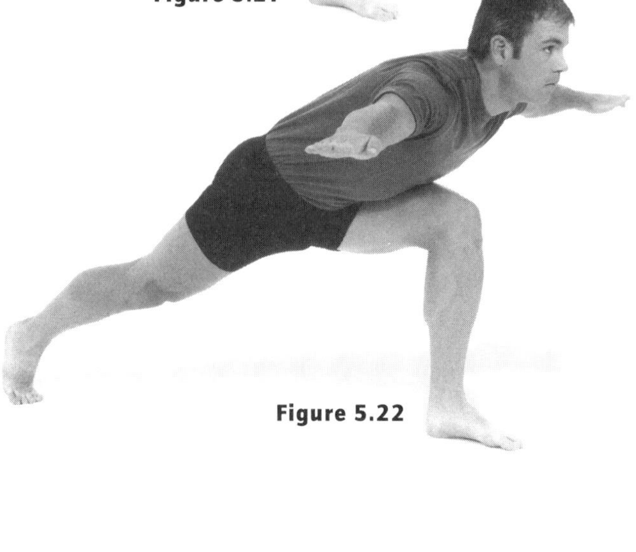

Figure 5.22

Hold your breath out for a moment.

Bring your left hand to the floor on the inside of your left leg. Breathe in and stretch your right arm straight up toward the ceiling (Figure 5.23). Look at your outstretched fingers and hold your breath in for a moment.

Breathe out, bring your arm down, swivel over to the right, and repeat the series facing right.

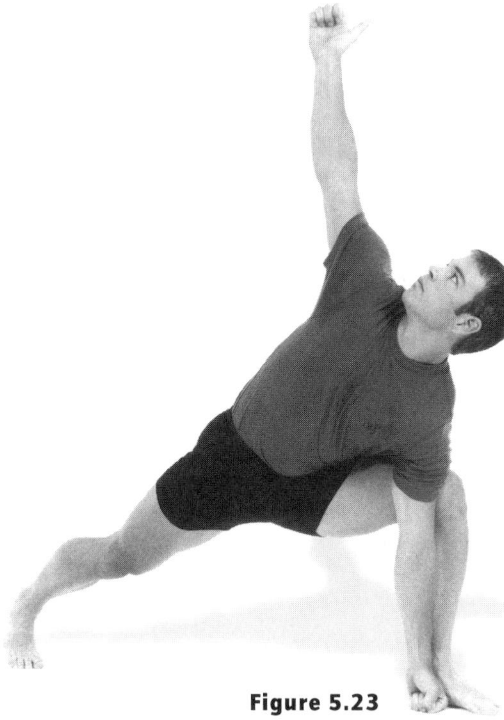

Figure 5.23

Spine Twist (pictured, pages 51–52)

Add the next two exercises between the Baby Pose and the Cobra Pose (pages 34–35). Sit up with both legs bent in front of you. Bend your left knee and lay it on the floor with your left foot under your right knee. Pick up your right foot and carry it across your left knee. Pull your left foot in close to your body.

Turn toward the right and bring your left arm over your right knee. With your left elbow, press your right knee back as far as it will comfortably go, then straighten your left arm and grasp the right big toe. If you can't reach your toe, grasp your ankle or knee instead.

Bring your right hand close in to your body, fingers pointed in, and straighten your arm. Straighten your back, breathe in looking forward, then breathe out as you twist toward the right as far as you can without straining. Look at a spot on the

wall just above eye level. Hold your breath out for a moment.

Release, and repeat on the opposite side.

Variation: for a less strenuous pose, keep the left leg outstretched.

Seated Sun Pose

Bring both legs straight out in front of you and flex your toes. Sit straight, breathe out with your arms at your sides (Figure 5.24), then breathe in as you raise your arms in a wide circle to the sides (Figure 5.25) and overhead. Press your palms together, look up, visualize the sun, and stretch from the rib cage (Figure 5.26).

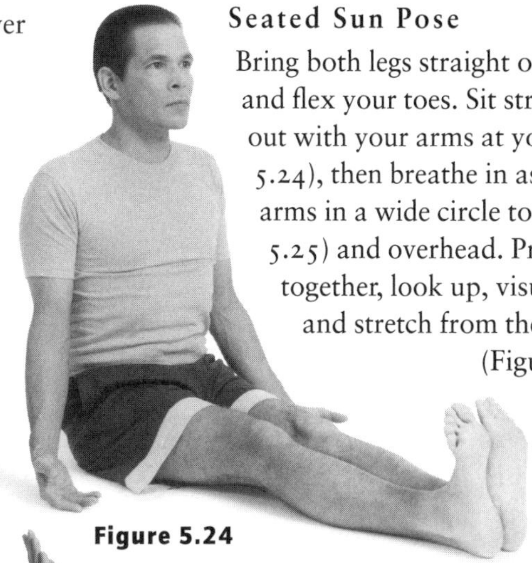

Figure 5.24

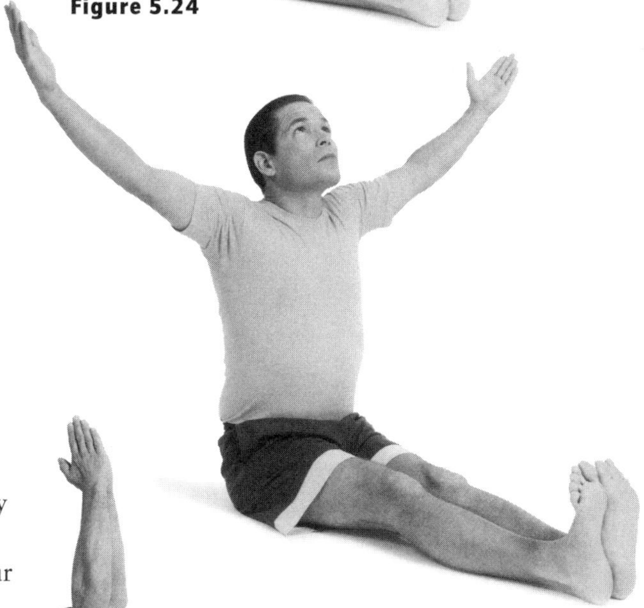

Figure 5.25

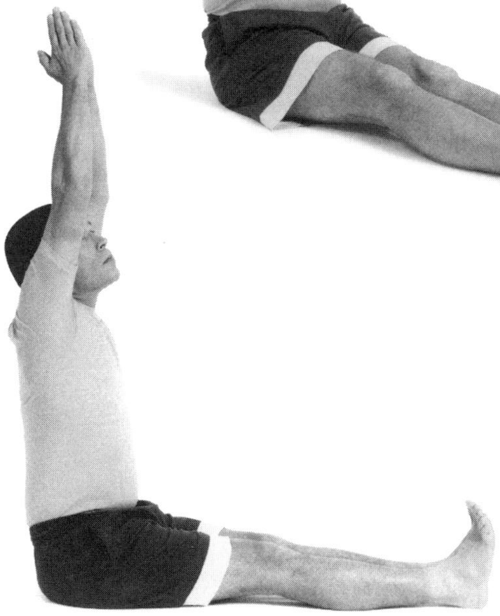

Figure 5.26

Hold your breath in for a moment.

Breathe out as you bend forward, tucking your chin toward your chest. Grasp your ankles, bend your elbows, and pull your torso toward your legs (remember to pull by bending your arms, not by pushing with your lower back). Hold your breath out for a moment.

If you are limber enough to reach your feet (and still bend your elbows), grasp your big toes as shown (Figures 5.27 and 5.28).

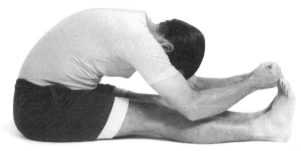

Figure 5.27

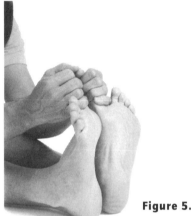

Figure 5.28

Release and breathe in, bringing your arms to the sides and over your head again. Stretch and look up as before. Breathe out and bring your arms back down to your sides. Repeat three times.

Boat Pose (pictured, page 75)

Add this exercise between the Cobra Pose and the Knee Squeeze (pages 35–36). Lying on your stomach, stretch your arms on the floor over your head and place your forehead on the floor. Breathe out. Breathe in as you lift your arms, legs, and head, looking up through your forehead. Hold your breath in for a moment. Breathe out and release, bringing your arms and forehead back to the floor. Repeat twice more.

Shoulder Stand (pictured, pages 75–76)

Add this exercise after the Knee Squeeze (page 36). Do not do this exercise if you have back or neck problems; substitute the Easy Bridge (page 78, Figures 5.54–5.55).

In a seated position with your knees bent and your arms around your knees, roll back and forth a few times, then roll back onto your shoulders, immediately supporting your back with your hands and keeping your knees bent and touching your forehead.

Slowly straighten your legs toward the ceiling and push your back straighter by using your hands. Stare at the spot between your big toes and breathe out. Hold your breath out for a moment. Breathe in and relax your breath.

Bring your knees back to your forehead, supporting your back with your hands, then roll forward into a cross-legged position, reaching your head and arms forward. Breathe naturally as you rest for at least 10 seconds.

Throwing Events: Discus, Javelin, Shot Put, Hammer

These sports date back to the earliest Olympiads, when the ability of a soldier to throw a weapon accurately at speed was crucial to survival. Throwing sports require balance, coordination, and upper-body strength. Yoga can help balance both sides of the body and provide overall flexibility and strength training. Breathing and fantasy techniques can improve focus.

Overuse of the shoulder can cause inflammation; great demands on the muscles of the back and lower body can contribute to muscle pulls and strains. The best way to prevent these injuries is thorough stretching of the upper body, especially the lower back.

Modify your core routine as follows:

Full Bend Variation

Add the next two exercises between the Neck Stretches and the Standing Sun Pose (pages 30–32). Stand with feet parallel. Clasp your hands behind your back. If you can, press your palms together (Figure 5.29). For an even greater stretch, lock your elbows so your shoulder blades are squeezed together. Breathe in and lift your arms in back as far

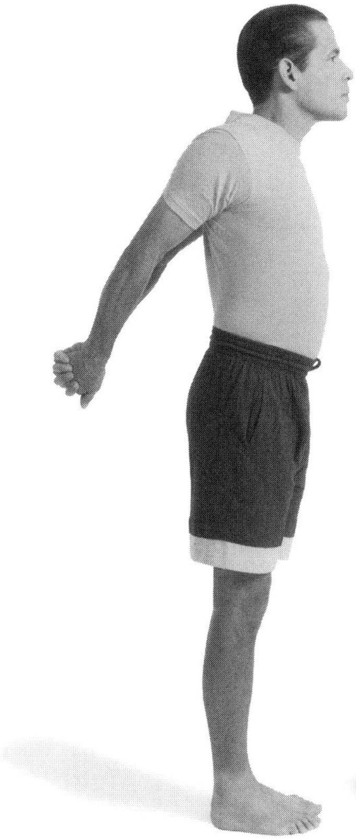

Figure 5.29 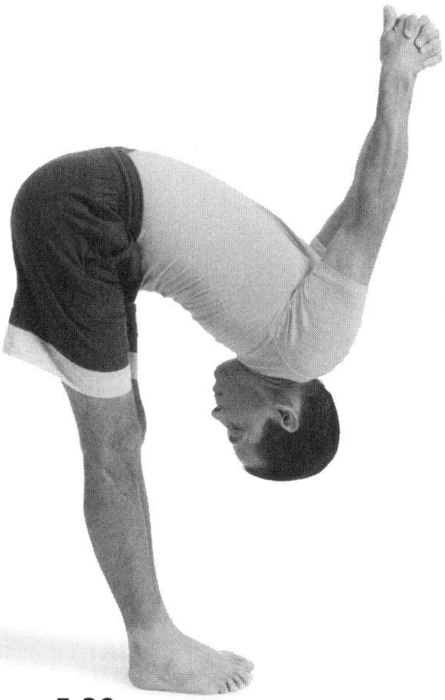   **Figure 5.30**

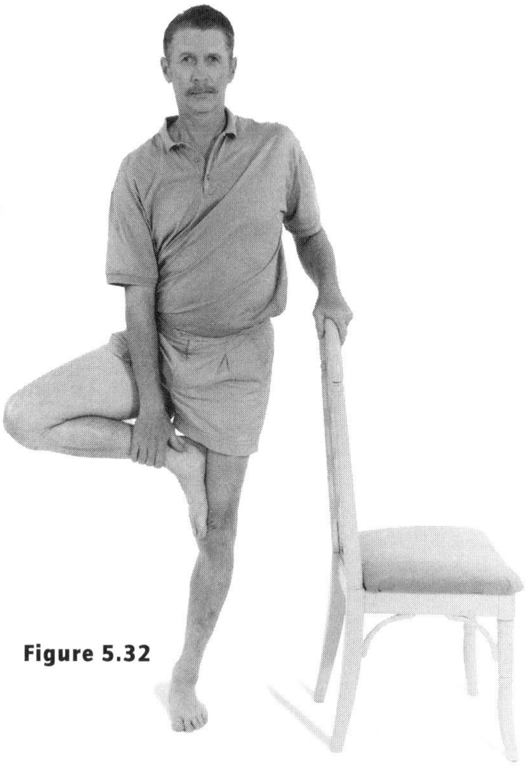

Figure 5.32

as you can without straining. Breathe out and bend forward, tucking your chin and keeping your arms in position (Figure 5.30). Hold your breath out for a moment. Breathe in and straighten. Repeat the exercise twice more.

Standing Reach and Twist

With feet parallel, breathe in and raise both your arms to the sides in a wide circle and overhead as high as possible without straining. Come up on your toes and stretch up toward the ceiling. Hold your breath in for a moment. Breathe out as you slowly lower your arms to your sides and your heels to the floor. Relax. Repeat twice more.

Breathe in again as before, lifting your heels and raising your arms overhead. Hold your breath in for a moment as you twist your upper body to the right (Figure 5.31).

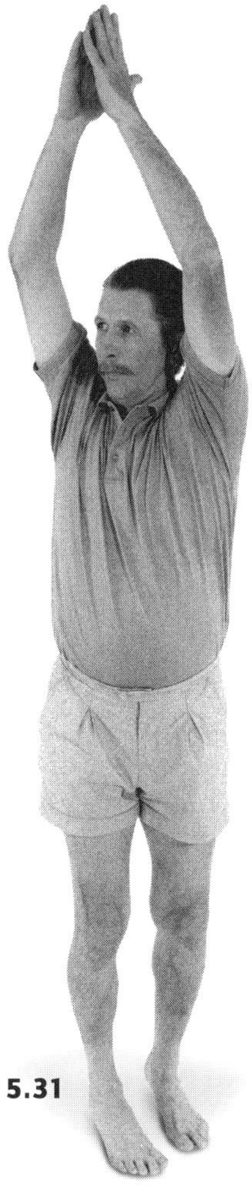

Figure 5.31

Twist back forward, breathe out, and lower your arms and heels. Repeat three times on each side.

Tree Pose

Add this exercise between the Standing Sun Pose and the Hip Rotation (pages 31–32). From a standing position, lift your right foot and place it on the inside of your left thigh (Figure 5.32). Relax the leg to help hold your foot in position. Bare feet will also help. If you feel unsteady, hold on to a sturdy chair. Steady yourself by gazing at one spot on the wall or floor without bending your neck. Breathe in as you raise your arms slowly over your head, straighten your arms, and place your palms together (Figure 5.33). Hold your breath in

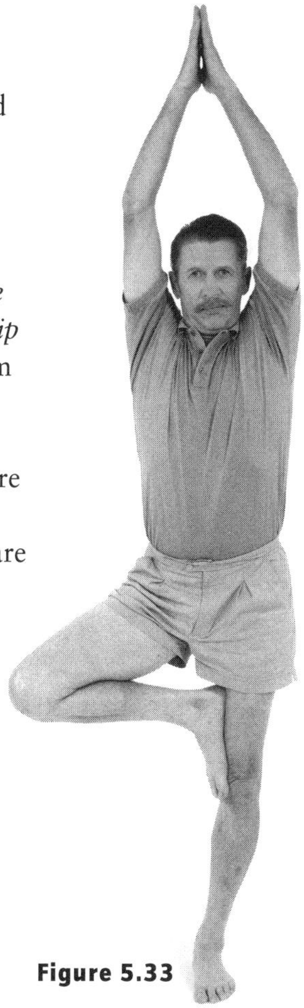

Figure 5.33

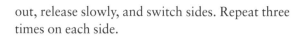

for a moment. Breathe out and bring your arms and leg down slowly. Repeat on the opposite side.

If you are limber enough, you may place your foot on top of your thigh for this exercise (Figure 5.34).

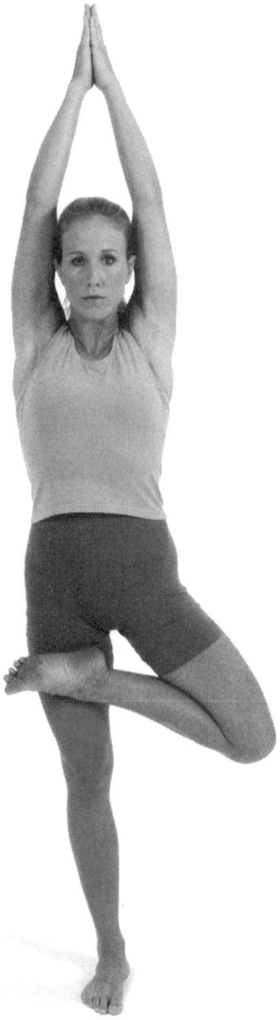

Figure 5.34

Bow Variation

Add the next two exercises between the Cat Breath and the Cobra V-Raise (page 34). Start on your hands and knees. Reach back with your left hand and grasp your right foot. Stare at one spot on the wall or floor for balance as you breathe in and lift your foot up and away from your body as far as possible (Figure 5.35). Hold your breath in for a moment. Breathe

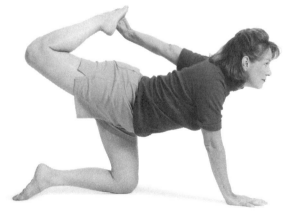

Figure 5.35

out, release slowly, and switch sides. Repeat three times on each side.

Camel Pose

From a kneeling position, separate your knees slightly, arch your back, and grasp your left heel with your left hand (Figure 5.36). Breathe normally. Do this once on each side to warm up. Then reach back and grasp both heels (Figure 5.37). Push your hips forward as far as possible without straining. Let your head gently fall back as you breathe out (unless you have a disk problem in your upper back or neck, in

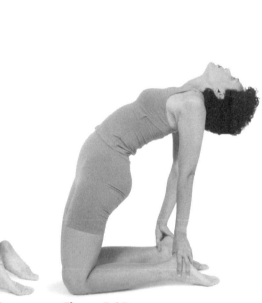

Figure 5.36   **Figure 5.37**

which case keep your head up). Breathe in and release. Rest.

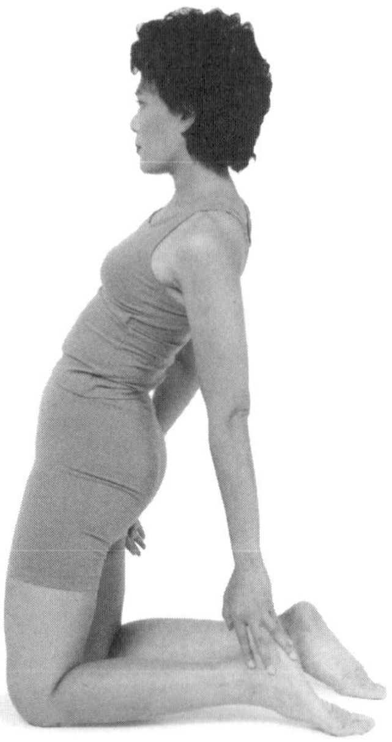

Variation: if you are unable to grasp both heels at once, do the exercise once on each side in the beginning position (Figure 5.36) instead.

Side Stretch

Add the next three exercises between the Baby Pose and the Cobra Pose (pages 34–35). Sit up in a comfortable cross-legged position. Breathe in, then breathe out as you lean to the right and stretch your left arm up over your head and toward the right, stretching the entire left side of your torso (Figure 5.38). Hold your breath out for a moment. Breathe in as you release, then repeat on the opposite side.

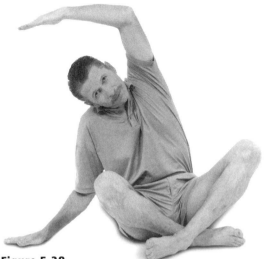

Figure 5.38

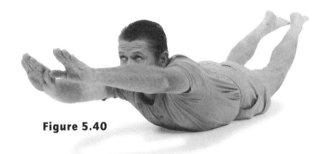

Figure 5.39

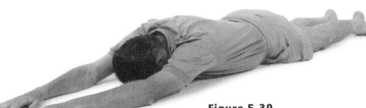

Figure 5.40

Plank Pose (pictured, page 78)

From a hands-and-knees position, straighten your legs out behind you, supporting yourself on your hands. Raise your hips and lower your shoulders until your body is in a straight line supported on your hands and feet. Shift your weight to your right arm and breathe in as you lift your left arm straight in front of you. Focus your gaze on your outstretched hand. Hold your breath in for a moment. Breathe out and release.

Still supporting yourself on your right arm, breathe in as you bring your left arm to the side and up toward the ceiling. This will twist your body to the left as well. Look up toward your hand. Hold your

breath in for a moment. Breathe out, bring your left hand down to the floor, and repeat the sequence on the opposite side. Then rest lying on your stomach.

Boat Pose

Lying on your stomach, stretch your arms on the floor over your head and place your forehead on the floor (Figure 5.39). Breathe out. Breathe in as you lift your arms, legs, and head, looking up through your forehead (Figure 5.40). Hold your breath in for a moment. Breathe out and release, bringing your arms and forehead back to the floor. Repeat twice more.

Shoulder Stand

Add the next two exercises after the Knee Squeeze (page 36). Do not do this exercise if you have back or neck problems; substitute the Easy Bridge (page 78, Figures 5.54–5.55).

In a seated position with your knees bent and your arms around your knees (Figure 5.41), roll back and forth a few times (Figure 5.42), then roll back onto your shoulders, immediately supporting your back with your hands (Figure 5.43) and keeping your knees bent and touching your forehead (Figure 5.44).

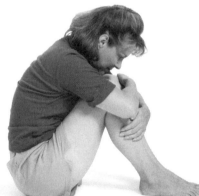

Figure 5.41

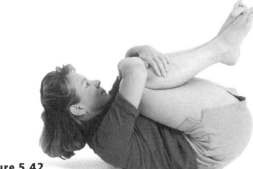

Figure 5.42

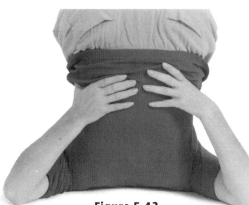

Figure 5.43

Slowly straighten your legs toward the ceiling and push your back straighter by using your hands (Figure 5.45). Stare at the spot between your big toes and breathe out. Hold

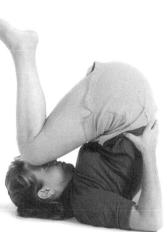

Figure 5.44

your breath out for a moment. Breathe in and relax your breath.

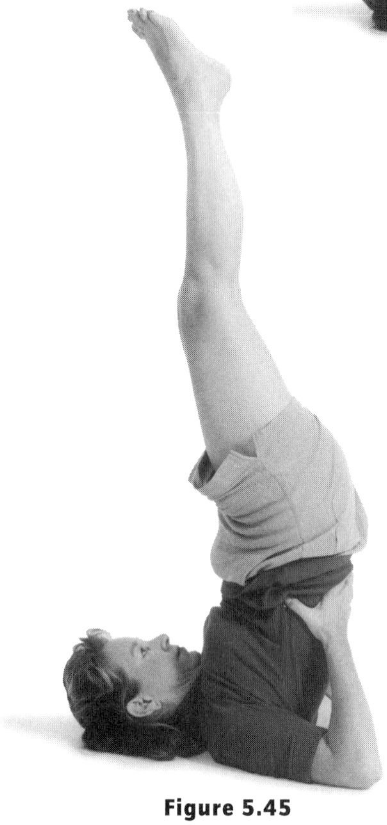

Bring your knees back to your forehead, supporting your back with your hands, then roll forward into a cross-legged position, reaching your head and arms forward (Figure 5.46). Breathe naturally as you rest for at least 10 seconds.

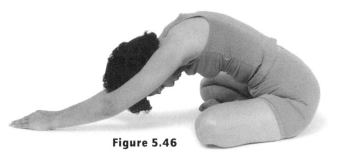

Figure 5.46

Humming Breath

Sit up in a comfortable position, either cross-legged or sitting on your feet, or sit on the edge of a chair with your hands on your knees. Breathe in completely just as you would in the Complete Breath, described on page 20. Now breathe out with an audible *hummmm* sound, making the tone steady and loud until your breath is gone—just like the sound of a bumblebee. Let the sound vibrate in your throat, and keep pushing with your belly muscles so that the sound doesn't trail off at the end. Try to keep the sound steady. Repeat several times.

Bowling

Bowling builds coordination and a good sense of timing and distance. Yoga can balance both sides of the body as well as stretch and strengthen the shoulders, legs, and back to help prevent injury.

Bowling demands the exact same movements of the body with every shot, so frequent play can lead to overuse injuries in the shoulder, back, and hip. The best way to prevent these injuries is through thorough stretching warm-up of the upper body, especially the back.

Modify your core routine as follows:

Full Bend

Add this exercise between the Neck Stretches and the Standing Sun Pose (pages 30–32). Stand with feet parallel, a few inches apart. Breathe out completely. Breathe in as you slowly raise your arms up and out to your sides, parallel to the floor (Figure 5.47). Stretch back a little as you hold your breath in for a moment, then breathe out as you slowly bend forward, leading with your hands, until you are as far forward as possible. Let your whole body go limp (Figure 5.48). Now breathe in and slowly come back up, bringing your arms out to the sides again. Continue breathing in as you straighten up and out as

Figure 5.45

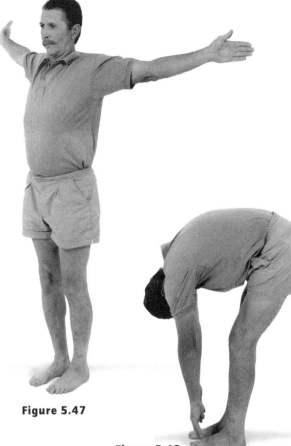

Figure 5.47

Figure 5.48

arm and your right leg. Breathe out and hold your breath out for a moment.

Breathe in and release. With your legs in the same position, breathe out as you stretch both arms out to the sides, resting your chest on your left thigh. Hold your breath out for a moment.

Bring your left hand to the floor on the inside of your left leg. Breathe in and stretch your right arm straight up toward the ceiling. Look at your outstretched fingers and hold your breath in for a moment.

Breathe out, bring your arm down, swivel over to the right, and repeat the series facing right.

Cat Variation

Add this exercise between the Cat Breath and the Cobra V-Raise (page 34). This sequence is done with a strong, steady breath pattern. On hands and knees, start by breathing in. Breathe out strongly as you round your back up and forward and bring your right knee to your forehead (Figure 5.49).

Breathe in briefly as you release that position and breathe out

Figure 5.49

you bend forward, matching your breath to your movement. Repeat several times.

Lunge Series (pictured, pages 70–71)

Add this exercise between the Twisting Triangle and the Cat Breath (pages 33–34). With your toes pointed inward, spread your legs as far apart as you comfortably can. Breathe in as you turn completely toward the left and bend your left leg, bringing your left elbow underneath your left knee and resting on both fists. Keep your right leg straight if you can; if that position is too strenuous, rest your knee on the floor. Bend your head toward the floor as you breathe out. Hold your breath out for a moment. Breathe in and release. Repeat on the opposite side.

Breathe in as you turn back to the left. Breathe out as you rest both elbows on the floor with your left elbow inside your left knee, lower your right knee to the floor, clasp your hands, and bend your head toward your hands. Hold your breath out for a moment.

Breathe in as you push yourself up, rest your left arm on your left thigh, and straighten your right

again strongly as you go into the next position. Straighten and lift your right leg in back, bend your elbows, and arch your back so your chin reaches toward the floor (Figure 5.50). Breathe in briefly as you release that position and breathe out as you go back to the first position (Figure 5.49) for

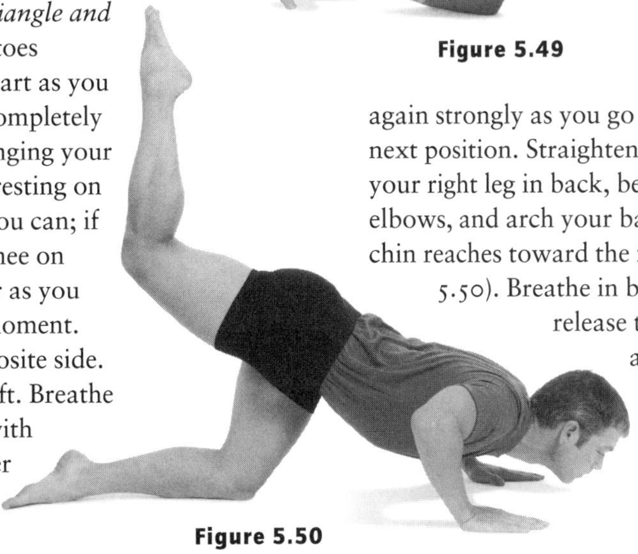

Figure 5.50

the next repetition. Repeat three to six times on each side, slowly.

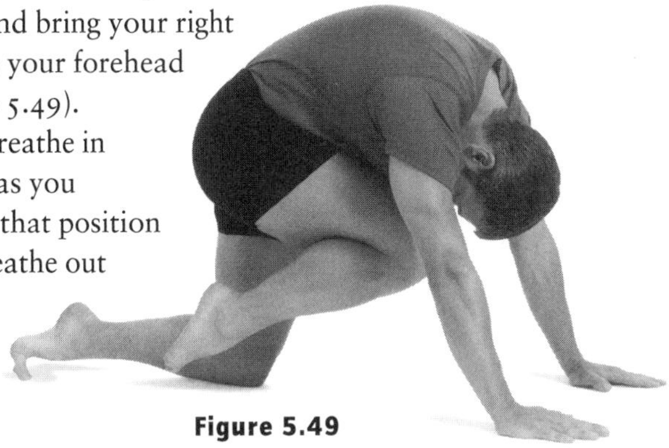

Plank Pose

Add this exercise between the Cobra V-Raise and the Baby Pose (pages 34–35). From a hands-and-knees position, straighten your legs out behind you, supporting yourself on your hands. Raise your hips and lower your shoulders until your body is in a straight line supported on your hands and feet (Figure 5.51). Shift your weight to your right arm and breathe in as you lift your left arm straight in front of you (Figure 5.52). Focus your gaze on your outstretched hand. Hold your breath in for a moment. Breathe out and release.

Still supporting yourself on your right arm, breathe in as you bring your left arm to the side and up toward the ceiling (Figure 5.53). This will twist your body to the left as well. Look up toward your hand. Hold your breath in for a moment. Breathe out, bring your left hand down to the floor, and repeat the sequence on the opposite side. Then rest lying on your stomach.

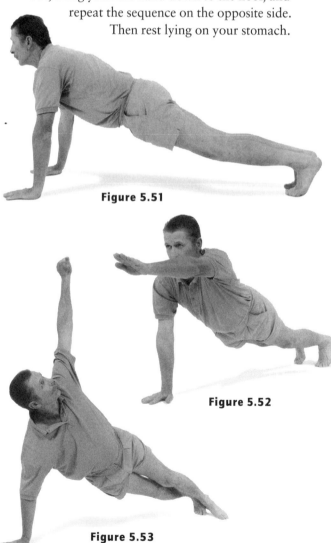

Figure 5.51

Figure 5.52

Figure 5.53

Side Stretch (pictured, page 75)

Add the next two exercises between the Baby Pose and the Cobra Pose (pages 34–35). Sit up in a comfortable cross-legged position. Breathe in, then breathe out as you lean to the right and stretch your left arm up over your head and toward the right, stretching the entire left side of your torso. Hold your breath out for a moment. Breathe in as you release, then repeat on the opposite side.

Boat Pose (pictured, page 75)

Lying on your stomach, stretch your arms on the floor over your head and place your forehead on the floor. Breathe out. Breathe in as you lift your arms, legs, and head, looking up through your forehead. Hold your breath in for a moment. Breathe out and release, bringing your arms and forehead back to the floor. Repeat twice more.

Easy Bridge

Add this exercise after the Knee Squeeze (page 36). Lying on your back, bend your knees and separate your legs and feet several inches; place your arms at your sides, palms down (Figure 5.54). Breathe in, then breathe out as you lift your hips, arching your back and tucking your chin into your chest (Figure 5.55). Hold your breath out for a moment. Repeat twice more.

Variation: if you are very limber, you can grasp your ankles with both hands.

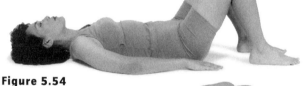

Figure 5.54

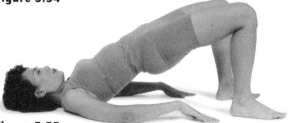

Figure 5.55

Golf

For a complete routine for golf, please see Chapter 4, pages 42–46.

6

ENDURANCE SPORTS

Running, Walking, Cycling, Triathlon, Cross-Country Skiing, Speed Skating, Swimming, In-Line Skating, Basketball, Soccer, Football, and Rugby

What I like least about triathlons is the high cost of entrance fees.

—Dale O'Hara

When I was racing, something else would push. There would be this surge, just like running a turbo engine. You get this turbo charge and you just get pushed into moving more and harder and faster and stronger, and it's incredibly exhilarating.

—Lea Jackson

Until I finished my first Ironman distance triathlon (2.4-mile swim, 112-mile bike ride, and 26.2-mile run), the only emotion I felt was either joy or sadness, depending on how I did. During the Ironman I went through many emotions: happiness, sadness, optimism, pessimism, crying, laughing. Then there were moments between all of these where I felt stillness—no thoughts, no pain, no environment, no race—just in the moment.

—Dale O'Hara

The strain of the extended demand of a marathon is relived every day for those athletes who drive themselves to their limit and beyond. When practiced competitively, the sports covered in this chapter have a similar theme: "How much can I take? How fast can I go while I am putting in my best effort? How long can I last?" The endurance aspects of speed events and team games such as football and basketball may not be obvious because they do not require continuous exertion. However, sprint events usually consist of a number of heats or repetitions that cumulatively demand endurance as much as speed, and even though team games have much more downtime than actual exertion, the games consist of any number of burst strength/speed exertion repetitions. Sport-specific training activities also take up a vast number of hours and often include pure endurance exertion.

Counteracting the tendency toward self-punishment for its own sake is the best way Yoga can work for you if you practice endurance sports. In Chapter 1, I mentioned the ethic of nonviolence. In talking to runners, cyclists, and cross-country skiers, I find a common habit: they brutally push their bodies to the point of pain, then try to pass that point into a feeling where the pain doesn't matter. This produces a change of consciousness in them that denies the pain of the physical and rests totally on the driving force of personal, egotistical will. Eventually this practice will cause deterioration in the body, because the body is signaling exhaustion and the personal ego-driven will of the athlete is demanding that it keep performing anyway.

This old "no pain, no gain" theory can be the cause of early burnout in a sport. This theory is not the classical sacrifice to sport that has been described in mythology. The body is sacrificed to the athlete's personal egotistic will, not used as a gift to the unknown inner spiritual force.

Although the injuries that force early retirement may not be seen in the body, they take a toll on the overall performance of the athlete. Eventually, unless extra support is given to the physical body, it breaks down. Most people use food or drug supplements to prevent this deterioration, but these substances will not ease the emotional upset caused by forcing the body to pain.

Current research on exercise and health has found an important connection between the intensity of exercise and susceptibility to disease. Most people are aware that moderate exercise can help bolster one's immune system and thus prevent infection. It is best to avoid intense, exhaustive training, though, which can actually deplete the immune system and raise the risk of infection.

I suggest that when you reach the point of pain in effort, try the concentrated breath exercise described in Chapter 5, page 62. Concentrated breath training will send support from the inner emotional/spiritual/power body to the physical body when it needs the extraordinary strength that is required to surpass its ordinary limits. The breathing technique forms a bridge for the inner emotional/spiritual/power body to operate in support of the physical. Instead of whipping the physical to perform, you can offer it help when it needs it.

I am sure you have noticed the uncanny ability of people in the grip of extreme emotion to exhibit tremendous strength. Everyone has heard stories, for instance, of mothers lifting a car off a child trapped in an accident. A similar phenomenon happens in sport when players lose themselves to the emotional grip of the game. Many times I have watched coaches call for a time-out as they realize the super strength that emerges at this time in an opponent. These coaches are aware that this emotional flowering brings with it tremendous strength. The emotional joining of the physical body is undependable, however; unless regular training is involved, it flashes at rare times.

The inner body is your source of power, and you can use breath concentration to call for its help when the physical body lags. It comes forward when called as a support; it is the primitive source of strength. When it expresses itself, the brutal demand

You sometimes think practice is tedious and boring, but then you remember that without practice and discipline, game time performance would most likely not be to its highest level. In practice I think about how this will help me improve and how pushing myself in practice will help my game. I would often push myself to pain and exhaustion and then stay over to practice serves or foul shots.

—Alice Kennedy

on the physical is removed. It comes to help, not to whip, the body. The physical body loves the feeling of it and sooner or later learns that it is always available. It never runs out. It is limitless.

Sometimes a discipline may be hard, fatiguing, or discouraging at first. There is an old saying, part of the well-known yogic text *The Bhagavad Gita*, which says: "Like poison in the beginning, like nectar in the end." This verse is referring to the disciplines of Yoga, which can be a little difficult when first begun, but soon lead to the sweet rewards of self-awareness, empowerment, and the satisfaction of knowing that you performed at your very best.

Whether you are training for a competition, or just working out to keep yourself in shape, the ideal attitude is to be running, or swimming, or cycling simply because you love it. Many people have talked and written about the experience known as runner's high, a feeling of euphoria, confidence, and loss of self that accompanies extended effort. Most athletes enjoy this experience in the physical self, but the classical athlete would offer these feelings to the inner body for expression.

I like cycling because it's a lot of fun. And again because it takes me places. It's not boring. But you can't pick the weather. I used to do it year-round when I was younger. But as I got older and more responsible, I had less time for it. If I was in good shape I probably would go day and night no matter what the weather. When I was younger I would even ride in the rain. Now I use it as an escape from my relatives when they come to visit!

—Peter Cerar, cyclist

Preventing Boredom

All endurance sports have one common problem: boredom in the constant daily training. Swimming seems most problematical. How long can you look at the bottom of a pool without some need for another view to give some relief from the monotony? At least in other endurance sports, such as running, the scenery changes.

There is no question that I use triathlons as an escape from unhappiness. However, I mostly think that I am searching for something. What that is I have no idea. My mother passed away when I was 20 years old and since that time I have expected nothing less than being my best in anything I do. I love to keep pushing the limit meter—to go further each day than I previously thought I could.

—Dale O'Hara

If you can find a way to add enjoyment to your training, you can look forward to your daily practice. The great challenge is how long and how fast you can do it, and the training of repetitive action is paramount to gaining the strength and ability to perform.

My suggestion for the relief of the monotony of daily work is to practice concentration on the breath while you train. This has an effect of drawing your mind into silence, and when this happens you will not feel bored. There is another side effect to this practice that is equally valuable: it supplies extraordinary energy. You will find yourself much less tired after training and more emotionally steady.

Many times people use sport as a relief from everyday stress. For instance, if you need a break from whatever you are doing, whether it is intense work or a difficult situation, you go out for a run. The problem with this strategy is that whatever was causing the stress that made you take the break usually remains carried along with you in your mind and emotions. Conversations, phone calls, business plans, family matters—all linger in the mind while you are taking that break. Sometimes Yoga students are able to bring their techniques into play to counteract this tendency, as illustrated by the statement of one of the athletes we interviewed:

The thing about swimming that I like so much is that I get really lost in it. There have been times when I get in the pool and I may be grousing about something or worried about something, and if I swim for more than 5 or 10 minutes I'm not thinking about anything. It really becomes kind of a meditative state. I don't have any recollection of thinking about anything.

Concentrating on your breath as you begin your activity takes only a minute or two. Then, as you start your run or other activity, it is easy to continue thinking of your breath. You become very aware of the sound and the feeling of your breathing. You can fantasize your lungs expanding and flooding your physical body with oxygen.

Concentrated awareness of your breath will put all other thought out of your mind. If you are emotionally upset when you begin your training, try practicing a few breath exercises. This breath practice will calm and soothe emotional upset by giving you a break from the upset that runs through your mind like a continuous-loop tape. This break from ordinary thought allows your inner body to become outwardly active. New strength will flood through you. You will find with practice that this breath concentration exercise will become automatic in your daily training as you continue to use it. Your body will love it and because of that, you will not feel resistance to everyday training.

Notice what you think about while you are doing your daily routine. You will find that the stress of your thought process will affect the stress felt by your physical body. The body gains more strength when mental stress is quieted, and breath concentration will do this. You will find that your mind is unable to run its normal pattern of talking to itself when concentrated on breath. This is very much like plugging a leak. The athletic body needs the approach of one-pointed attention. When your attention becomes scattered, you lose your strength and ability.

After a $1,000 alignment on the car and still no improvement in my winnings, I found myself at a race in Sebring, the first ever solo trials in Florida. I was very nervous and noticed my breath was uneven, so I reminded myself of my breathing exercises and calmed my breath with several deep complete breaths. Sitting in my car, all strapped in with my helmet on, sweating in the Florida heat, I got very quiet, almost like during meditation. I realized that I knew perfectly well how to drive the car, I knew when to turn and how to apply the gas smoothly, late apexes, and all that fancy talk racers like to throw around. That is when I decided to relax and let something that I knew was inside me have a crack at it. I was still driving, but it was sort of like I was feeling how to do it instead of thinking my way through it.

I was dripping wet with perspiration when my turn finally came. The starter waved the green flag, the car took off, and I was along for a really thrilling ride. I actually was the fastest full-bodied car that day, getting quicker each time I went out. But the best part was that there was an almost magical feeling that went with it.

I kept on relaxing and feeling my way around the track and went on to win the state championship, the regional championship, the solo trials championship, and the Solo 1 Sebring Championship that year.

—David Wilson

GLYCOGEN LOADING FOR LONG-DISTANCE FUEL

"Hitting the wall" is caused by running out of muscle fuel. Many endurance athletes benefit from maximizing glycogen stores before an event of continuous exertion lasting more than $1^{1}/_{2}$ hours. Try saturating your stores of fuel by following this program:

1. One week before the event, try to get 70 percent of total calories from starches.

2. Every other day cut your training effort by half.
3. Rest the day before the event.
4. Top off glycogen stores with a high-carbohydrate, low-sugar, low-fat, and low-fiber meal three to four hours before the event.

The Sport Routines

The exercise routines recommended for endurance sports provide overall strengthening and limbering benefits for the large muscle groups. Balance exercises are included to build strength as well as the mental steadiness needed for endurance events. A breathing technique, the Complete Breath with Arm Circles, is included in each routine here to build stamina and improve breath capacity. For best results, always include a few minutes of meditation in your practice session.

> *Tennis is a part of me and I do not consider it just a sport. When I have not been able to play in the past because of injuries, work, etc., I missed it very much. I do not drink, smoke, or take drugs—maybe because I am addicted to tennis instead! It definitely releases stress, which is essential in my business, being that it gives me a better quality of life. I have more energy for my family, work, etc.*
>
> *I have always believed that you do not learn anything from a win—only a loss. Some of my past losses have triggered a lot of positive changes in my training and game.*
>
> —Marsha Wolak

Running/Walking

Running and walking provide excellent heart/lung conditioning, and are among the fastest ways to lose fat. However, running places extreme stress on knee joints. Muscles and ligaments in the spine and back of the legs tend to tighten, possibly cramp, due to constant contraction. Walking places less stress on the joints, but leg and back muscles can also tighten without proper stretching to compensate. Yoga exercises will stretch and strengthen leg and hip muscles, improve the strength and flexibility of the spine, and improve stamina by increasing breath capacity. Runners are vulnerable to abnormal eating patterns; see sidebar on page 127 for recommendations.

Most running and walking injuries are due to chronic overuse of the ankle, knee, foot, hip, and back. Sometimes back or leg pain can be caused by physical abnormalities such as having one leg longer than the other. The best way to prevent these injuries is through stretching and strengthening of all the leg and back muscles and joints.

Modify your core routine as follows:

Complete Breath with Arm Circles

Add this exercise before the Shoulder Roll (pages 28–29). Sit in a comfortable position as described in Chapter 2, page 20. Begin the Complete Breath exercise, but add this component: as you breathe in, raise your arms in circles to the sides and over your head. At the top, hold your breath in for just a moment as you stretch up with your fists (Figure 6.1). Then breathe out as you lower your arms in a circle back to the floor. Repeat three to five times.

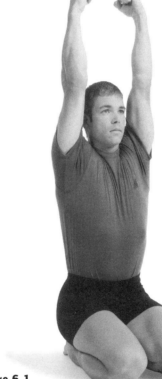

Figure 6.1

Leg Raises (pictured, page 103)

Add the next four exercises between the Neck Stretches and the Standing Sun Pose (pages 30–32). Stand straight with both hands on hips. (If you feel unsteady, you can hold on to a chair with your right hand.) Breathe out completely. Breathe in as you lift your right leg straight up in front as high as possible without bending your knee or straining. Hold the position and your breath for a moment. Breathe out and lower your leg. Breathe in and lift your right leg straight out to the side as far as possible without straining. Hold the position and your breath for a moment. Breathe out and lower your leg. Breathe in and lift your right leg straight out in back as far as possible without bending your knee. Hold the position and your breath for a moment. Breathe out and lower your leg. Repeat with your left leg.

Standing Knee Squeeze
(pictured, page 89)
Breathe in as you lift and bend your right knee and wrap both arms around it. Hold your breath in as you squeeze the knee to your chest and bend your forehead toward your knee. Repeat three times on each side.

Variation: if your balance is unsteady, hold on to a sturdy chair or counter for support with one hand.

Dancer Pose and Extension
From a standing position, bend your left leg back and grasp your left foot with your right hand (Figure 6.2). Throughout the exercise, steady yourself by fixing your gaze on one spot on the wall in front of you. Slowly move into the completed Dancer Pose by raising your left arm straight up toward the ceiling and pulling your lifted leg up and back as far as possible without strain (Figure 6.3). Keep your right (supporting) leg straight and keep your gaze focused on one spot. Breathe in and hold your breath in for a moment.

Maintaining your gaze, slowly breathe out and lower your body into the extended position (Figure 6.4). Keep your lifted leg as far up and back as possible. Your left arm extends straight ahead. Your supporting leg remains straight. Stare at one spot for balance. Don't strain. Hold for a moment, then breathe in, come back to a standing position, and switch sides.

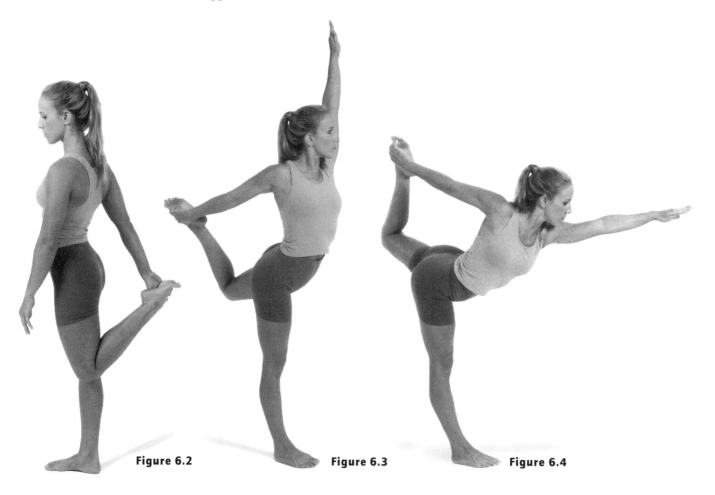

Figure 6.2   Figure 6.3   Figure 6.4

Eagle Pose

Stare at one spot on the wall or floor for balance. Bend your right leg slightly. Wrap your left leg over and behind the right leg (Figure 6.5; if you can't reach behind the leg, just go as far as you can). When you're steady, bend your torso and place your right elbow on your left knee (Figure 6.6). Then place your left elbow inside your right elbow, turn your hands toward each other, and clasp your fingers. Breathe out as you bend your head so your forehead rests on your hands (Figure 6.7). Hold your breath out for a moment. Slowly breathe in, untwist, and switch sides.

Variation: lace your fingers behind your back. If you can, lock your elbows, squeezing your shoulder blades together. Lift one leg as high as possible, bend your supporting leg, rest your chest on your thigh if possible, and lift your arms away from your back. Breathe out and hold for a moment. Release and switch sides.

Lunge Series (pictured, page 90)

With your toes pointed inward, spread your legs as far apart as you comfortably can. Breathe in as you turn completely toward the left and bend your left leg, bringing your left elbow underneath your left knee and resting on both fists. Keep your right leg straight if you can; if that position is too strenuous, rest your knee on the floor. Bend your head toward the floor as you breathe out. Hold your breath out for a moment. Breathe in and release. Repeat on the opposite side.

Breathe in as you turn back to the left. Breathe out as you rest both elbows on the floor with your left elbow inside your left knee, lower your right knee to the floor, clasp your hands, and bend your head toward your hands. Hold your breath out for a moment.

Breathe in as you push yourself up, rest your left arm on your left thigh, and straighten your right arm and your right leg. Breathe out and hold your breath out for a moment.

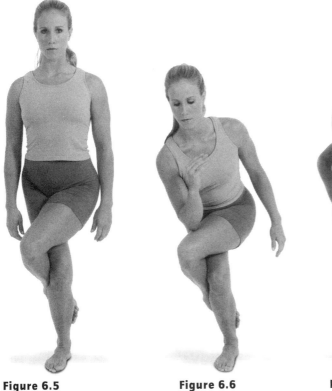

Figure 6.5   **Figure 6.6**   **Figure 6.7**

Breathe in and release. With your legs in the same position, breathe out as you stretch both arms out to the sides, resting your chest on your left thigh. Hold your breath out for a moment.

Warrior Pose (pictured, page 110)

Add the next two exercises between the Twisting Triangle and the Cat Breath (pages 33–34). Place both hands on your right knee and lift your left leg straight in back. Bend your right knee and let your torso rest on your right thigh as you slide your hands down to support either side of your right ankle. Keep your left leg high in back. Tuck your head. Breathe out and hold your breath out for a moment. Breathe in, slowly release, and repeat on opposite side.

Bring your left hand to the floor on the inside of your left leg. Breathe in and stretch your right arm straight up toward the ceiling. Look at your outstretched fingers and hold your breath in for a moment.

Breathe out, bring your arm down, swivel over to the right, and repeat the series facing right.

Seated Sun Pose and Alternate

Add the next two exercises between the Baby Pose and the Cobra Pose (pages 34–35). Bring both legs straight out in front of you and flex your toes. Sit straight, breathe out with your arms at your sides (Figure 6.8), then breathe in as you raise your arms in a wide circle to the sides (Figure 6.9) and over-head. Press your palms together, look up, visualize the sun, and stretch from the rib cage (Figure 6.10). Hold your breath in for a moment.

Breathe out as you bend forward, tucking your chin toward your chest. Grasp your ankles, bend your elbows, and pull your torso toward your legs (remember to pull by bending your arms, not by pushing with your lower back). Hold your breath out for a moment.

If you are limber enough to reach your feet (and still bend your elbows), grasp your big toes as shown (Figures 6.11 and 6.12).

Release and breathe in, bringing your arms to the sides and over your head again. Stretch and look up as before. Breathe out and bring your arms back down to your sides. Repeat three times.

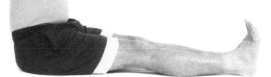

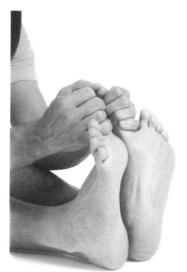

Figure 6.10

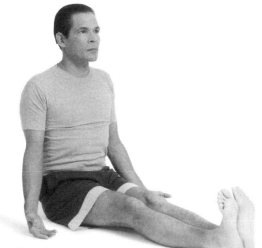

Figure 6.8

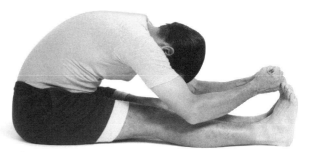

Figure 6.11

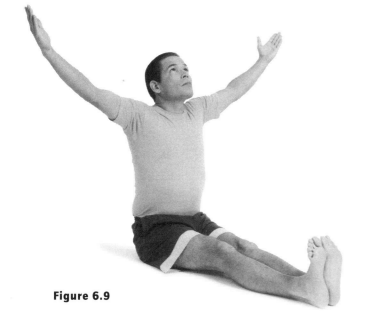

Figure 6.9

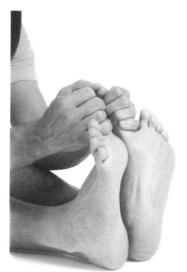

Figure 6.12

Alternate Seated Sun Pose: sit with legs outstretched. Bend your left knee and place your foot on the inside of your right thigh (Figure 6.13). Breathe in and bring your arms in a wide circle to the sides and over your head (Figure 6.14). Stretch from the rib cage and look up. Hold your breath in for a moment. Breathe out and bend forward over your outstretched leg, keeping your toes flexed. Grasp your ankle or foot with both hands, bend your elbows, and pull your torso gently toward your left

leg (Figure 6.15). Hold your breath out for a moment. *Note:* if you are limber enough to reach your foot and still bend your elbows, grasp the big toe with both hands, as shown (Figure 6.16).

Breathe in and raise your arms to the sides and over your head again. Stretch and look up. Hold your breath in for a moment Breathe out and lower. Repeat three times. Repeat on the opposite side.

Note: if you are limber enough so that your bent knee touches the floor when you place your foot on top of the opposite thigh instead of inside, you may do the exercise in this position. To increase limberness in your knee and hip, place your foot on top of the opposite thigh and gently press down on the upraised knee with your hand (Figure 6.17). Support yourself by leaning on your opposite hand, as shown.

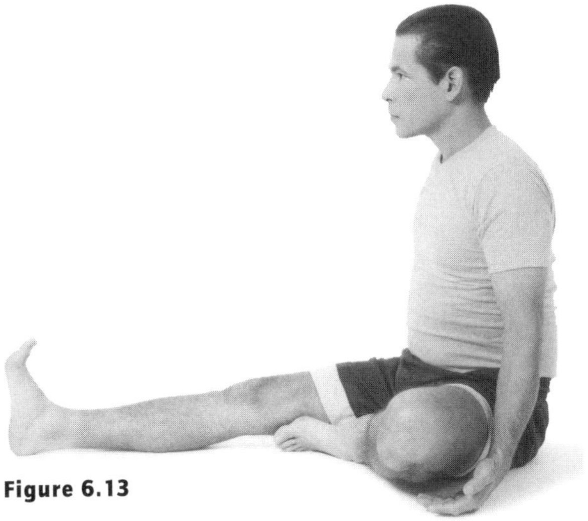

Figure 6.13

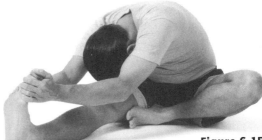

Figure 6.15

Figure 6.16

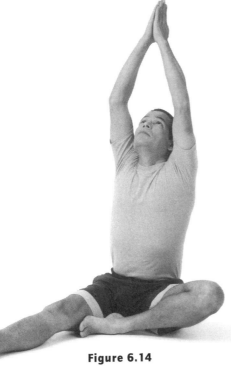

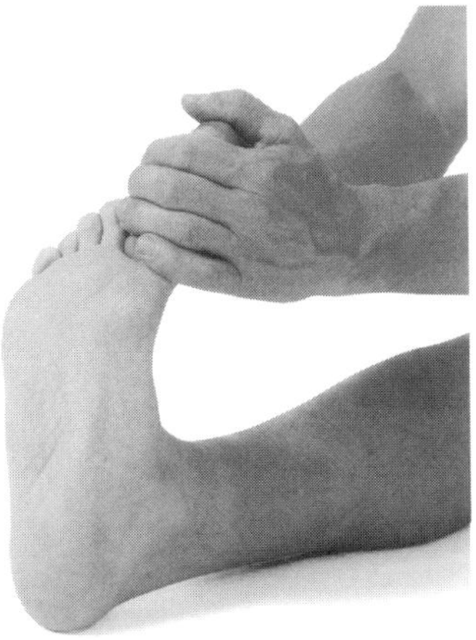

Figure 6.14

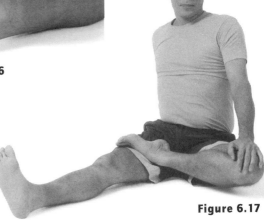

Figure 6.17

Bow Pose (pictured, page 94)

Lie on your stomach with your forehead to the floor. Bend your knees and grasp your ankles or feet with your hands (you may have to separate your legs slightly to reach). Breathe in as you lift and look up, pulling up on your feet so you balance on your stomach. Look up through your forehead. Visualize yourself as a bow. Hold your breath in for a moment. Breathe out and release. Repeat twice more.

Plow Pose (pictured, pages 97–98)

Add this exercise after the Knee Squeeze (page 36). From a seated position, bend your knees and roll back and forth once or twice. Then roll back onto your shoulders, bringing your knees to your forehead and supporting your back with your hands. Breathe in, hold a moment, then breathe out, extending your legs behind your head, carefully trying to touch your toes to the floor. Breathe naturally and hold the position for about 10 seconds.

If you wish, try this variation: straighten your arms on the floor over your head and hold for several seconds.

Breathe in and bend your knees back to your forehead, supporting your back with your hands,

When I did a lot of heavy cycling I relied heavily on Yoga to help me reach my goals. I used breathing and meditation for the focus, and I used stretching, the physical aspect of it, for avoiding injuries. When I've been cycling for awhile, I have a spring in my step. I think it takes away some of the "boogies" associated with stress and fatigue. It just makes me feel better.

When I bicycled regularly I would eat dinner before I went out to dinner because I couldn't afford to buy dinner for two for myself! I weighed only a hundred and fifty-four pounds. Cyclists who train burn more calories than any other sport I know. I remember reading that, where football players might burn three or four thousand calories a day, and lumberjacks probably the same, cyclists burn eight thousand calories daily.

—Peter Cerar

then roll forward to a cross-legged position, stretching your head and arms forward. Breathe naturally as you rest for about ten minutes.

Note: if you have a disk problem in your neck or upper back, do not do this exercise; substitute the Easy Bridge (page 78).

Cycling

Cycling provides a good cardiovascular workout that is easy on the joints. Yoga can add strengthening exercises for back and legs, plus limbering exercises for the spine, which is constantly bent forward when cycling. Breathing and meditation techniques will help improve concentration and stamina.

Overuse injuries from cycling include inflamed knee and Achilles' tendons and kneecap pain. Back pain can result from a poorly fitted bicycle. The best way to prevent these injuries is to stretch and strengthen the legs, knees, and back.

Modify your core routine as follows:

Complete Breath with Arm Circles (pictured, page 83)

Add this exercise before the Shoulder Roll (pages 28–29). Sit in a comfortable position as described in Chapter 2, page 20. Begin the Complete Breath exercise, but add this component: as you breathe in, raise your arms in circles to the sides and over your head. At the top, hold your breath in for just a moment as you stretch up with your fists. Then breathe out as you lower your arms in a circle back to the floor. Repeat three to five times.

Standing Knee Squeeze

Add the next two exercises between the Neck Stretches and the Standing Sun Pose (pages 30–32). Breathe in as you lift and bend your right knee and wrap both arms around it (Figure 6.18). Hold your breath in as you squeeze the knee to your chest and bend your forehead toward it. Repeat three times on each side.

Variation: if your balance is unsteady, hold on to a sturdy chair or counter for support with one hand (Figure 6.19).

Full Bend Variation (pictured, page 106)

Stand with your feet parallel. Clasp your hands behind your back. If you can, press your palms

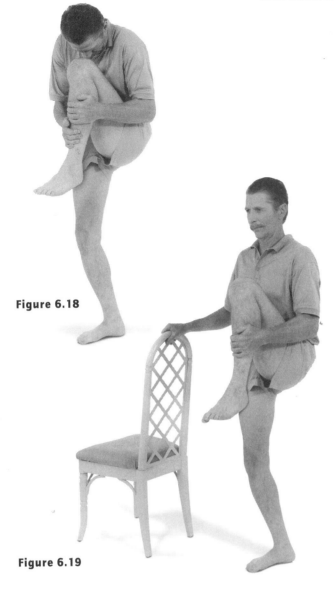

Figure 6.18

Figure 6.19

on the knee of your supporting leg. Keep your right (supporting) leg straight. Your torso and left leg should be in a straight line parallel to the floor. Keep your neck straight, breathe naturally, and look at a spot on the floor.

When you feel steady, release your grip on the support and place your palms together, pushing your arms out parallel to the floor. Relax your breath. Look forward at your hands. Lower your leg and return to a standing position. Rest until your breath returns to normal. Repeat on the opposite side.

Knee Bends

From the T Pose position, breathing naturally, keep your torso and lifted leg straight and parallel to the floor and, clasping your hands behind your back, gently bend your right knee and straighten (Figure 6.20). Try to do this without letting your shoulders and head bend toward the floor while your knee is bent. Keep breathing naturally. Stand up and rest. Repeat up to three times. Repeat on the opposite side.

Lunge Series

Add this exercise between the Cat Breath and the Cobra V-Raise (page 34). With your toes pointed inward, spread your legs as far apart as you comfortably can. Breathe in as you turn completely toward the left and bend your left leg, bringing your left elbow underneath your left knee and resting on both fists (Figure 6.21). Keep your right leg straight if you can; if that position is too strenuous, rest your knee on the floor. Bend your head toward the floor as you

together. For an even greater stretch, lock your elbows so your shoulder blades are squeezed together. Breathe in and lift your arms in back as far as you can without straining. Breathe out and bend forward, tucking your chin and keeping your arms in position. Hold your breath out for a moment. Breathe in and straighten. Repeat the exercise twice more.

T Pose (pictured, page 99)

Add the next two exercises between the Twisting Triangle and the Cat Breath (pages 33–34). When you are first learning this position, stand three to four feet from a chair or other support. Lean forward and hold on to the support with both hands. Lift your left leg in back as high as you can, ideally, parallel to the floor. Alternatively, brace yourself with both hands

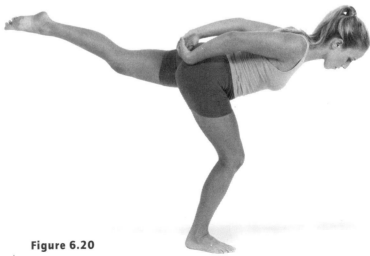

Figure 6.20

breathe out. Hold your breath out for a moment. Breathe in and release. Repeat on the opposite side.

Breathe in as you turn back to the left. Breathe out as you rest both elbows on the floor with your left elbow inside your left knee, lower your right knee to the floor, clasp your hands, and bend your head toward your hands (Figure 6.22). Hold your breath out for a moment.

Breathe in as you push yourself up, rest your left arm on your left thigh, and straighten your right arm and your right leg (Figure 6.23). Breathe out and hold your breath out for a moment.

Breathe in and release. With your legs in the same position, breathe out as you stretch both arms out to the sides, resting your chest on your left thigh (Figure 6.24). Hold your breath out for a moment.

Bring your left hand to the floor on the inside of your left leg. Breathe in and stretch your right arm straight up toward the ceiling (Figure 6.25). Look at your outstretched fingers and hold your breath in for a moment.

Breathe out, bring your arm down, swivel over to the right, and repeat the series (Figures 6.21–6.25) facing right.

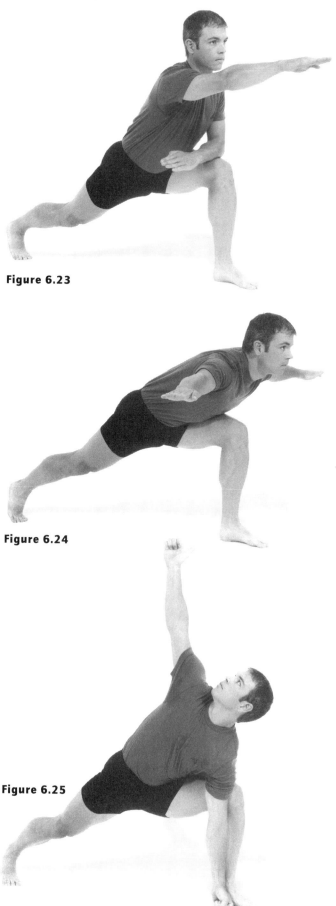

Figure 6.23

Figure 6.24

Figure 6.25

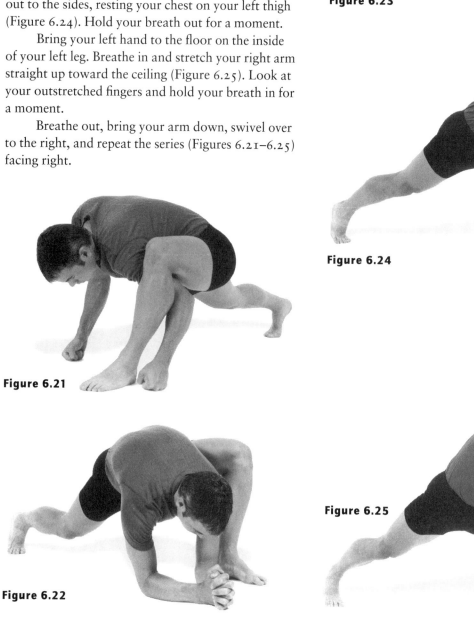

Figure 6.21

Figure 6.22

Camel Pose

Add the next five exercises between the Baby Pose and the Cobra Pose (pages 34–35). From a kneeling position, separate your knees slightly, arch your back, and grasp your left heel with your left hand (Figure 6.26). Breathe normally. Do this once on each side to warm up. Then reach back and grasp both heels (Figure 6.27). Push your hips forward as far as possible without straining. Let your head gently fall back as you breathe out (unless you have a disk problem in your upper back or neck, in which case keep your head up). Breathe in and release. Rest.

Variation: if you are unable to grasp both heels at once, do the exercise once on each side in the beginning position instead.

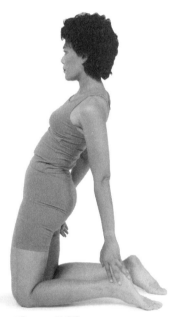

Figure 6.26   **Figure 6.27**

Pigeon Pose (pictured, page 100)

From a kneeling position, slide your right leg back so you are sitting on your left foot. Your right leg should be as straight as possible, knee to the floor. Place your hands on either side of your left knee and your forehead on the floor. Breathe out completely, then breathe in as you curl up, head first, then chest, then stomach, curling back as far as you can. You can press up on your fingertips for an extra stretch. Look up toward your forehead. Hold your breath in for a moment. Breathe out and curl down, stomach first, keeping your head and eyes up until your head reaches the floor. Repeat three times.

Then push yourself up on your fists, straighten your arms, relax your back, and stare at one spot on the floor about three feet in front of you. Breathe out and hold. Breathe in as you release the position.

Alternate Seated Sun Pose (pictured, page 87)

Sit with legs outstretched. Bend your left knee and place your foot on the inside of your right thigh. Breathe in and bring your arms in a wide circle to the sides and over your head. Stretch from the rib cage and look up. Hold your breath in for a moment. Breathe out and bend forward over your outstretched leg, keeping your toes flexed. Grasp your ankle or foot with both hands, bend your elbows, and pull your torso gently toward your left leg. Hold your breath out for a moment. (*Note:* if you are limber enough to reach your foot and still bend your elbows, grasp the big toe with both hands, as shown on page 87.)

Breathe in and raise your arms to the sides and over your head again. Stretch and look up. Hold your breath in for a moment. Breathe out and lower. Repeat three times. Repeat on the opposite side.

Note: if you are limber enough so that your bent knee touches the floor when you place your foot on top of the opposite thigh instead of inside, you may do the exercise in this position. To increase limberness in your knee and hip, place your foot on top of the opposite thigh and gently press down on the upraised knee with your hand. Support yourself by leaning on your opposite hand.

Side Stretch (pictured, page 112)

Sit in a comfortable cross-legged position. Breathe in, then breathe out as you lean to the right and stretch your left arm up over your head and toward the right, stretching the entire left side of your torso. Hold your breath out for a moment. Breathe in as you release, then repeat on the opposite side.

Bow Pose (pictured, page 94)

Lie on your stomach with your forehead to the floor. Bend your knees and grasp your ankles or feet with your hands (you may have to separate your legs slightly to reach). Breathe in as you lift and look up,

Soccer is definitely a young person's sport. It puts a lot of pressure on your legs. After college I was trying out for a semi-pro soccer team. They had watched our college team play and asked me to play for them.

So the first time I went to try out with their team it was on a lousy field. I was running and stepped in a hole at full speed. My knee crunched back in and that was it. I was a senior in college then and thought that my body was invincible. In a week or two the swelling went down a little bit and I went out and played basketball and it wrenched again. I did play again by going to college one more year in Canada. I found out you can play five years of college soccer in Canada as opposed to four years in the States. So I signed up for the college and took five courses and played college soccer one more season. My knee had recovered at that point. And then in Vermont I tried playing some again after that and wrenched my other knee out of place. So that was that. With two bad legs you're definitely out of it.

— Artie Guerin

[*Author's note:* despite these injuries, Artie went on to build a very successful career in tennis.]

pulling up on your feet so you balance on your stomach. Look up through your forehead. Visualize yourself as a bow. Hold your breath in for a moment. Breathe out and release. Repeat twice more.

Soccer, Football, and Rugby

These intense team sports require great stamina, agility, and strength. Yoga exercises can provide a good all-around stretching and strengthening routine; breathing and meditation can improve stamina and reaction time as well as the intuitive communication needed for team play.

Players are vulnerable to leg and back injuries due to contact (football and rugby) and high kicks (soccer), as well as leg, ankle, and foot injuries from pulled muscles resulting from constant motion in different directions. The best way to prevent these injuries is through solid stretching and strengthening of the legs and back.

Modify your core routine as follows:

Complete Breath with Arm Circles (pictured, page 83)

Add this exercise before the Shoulder Roll (pages 28–29). Sit in a comfortable position as described in Chapter 2, page 20. Begin the Complete Breath exercise, but add this component: as you breathe in, raise your arms in circles to the sides and over your head. At the top, hold your breath in for just a moment as you stretch up with your fists. Then breathe out as you lower your arms in a circle back to the floor. Repeat three to five times.

Windmill

Add this exercise between the Hip Rotation and the Side Triangle (pages 32–33). Keep your hands and feet in position after the Hip Rotation (Figure 6.28). Knees should remain straight but not locked throughout the movement. Breathe in and swivel toward the right, then breathe out as you bend your head toward your right knee (Figure 6.29) and across to your left knee. Start to breathe in as you lift up to a standing position (Figure 6.30), facing left, and swivel to the right to begin your second repetition. Repeat three to six times to the right, then three to six times to the left.

Lunge Series (pictured, page 90)

Add this exercise between the Cat Breath and the Cobra V-Raise (page 34). With your toes pointed inward, spread your legs as far apart as you comfortably can. Breathe in as you turn completely toward the left and bend your left leg, bringing your left elbow underneath your left knee and resting on both fists. Keep your right leg straight if you can; if that position is too strenuous, rest your knee on the floor. Bend your head toward the floor as you breathe out. Hold your breath out for a moment. Breathe in and release. Repeat on the opposite side.

Breathe in as you turn back to the left. Breathe out as you rest both elbows on the floor with your left elbow inside your left knee, lower your right knee to the floor, clasp your hands, and bend your

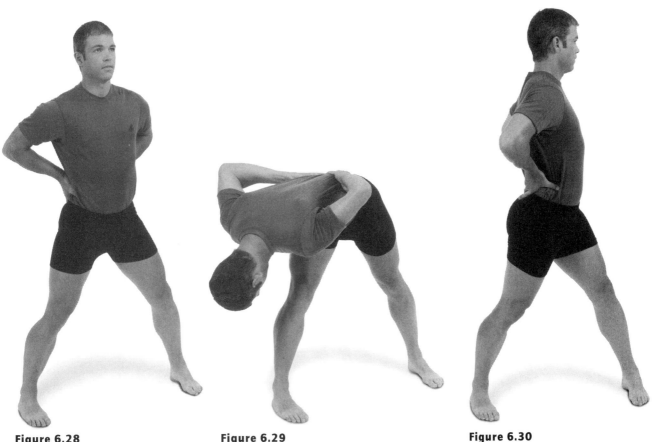

Figure 6.28   **Figure 6.29**   **Figure 6.30**

head toward your hands. Hold your breath out for a moment.

Breathe in as you push yourself up, rest your left arm on your left thigh, and straighten your right arm and your right leg. Breathe out and hold your breath out for a moment.

Breathe in and release. With your legs in the same position, breathe out as you stretch both arms out to the sides, resting your chest on your left thigh. Hold your breath out for a moment.

Bring your left hand to the floor on the inside of your left leg. Breathe in and stretch your right arm straight up toward the ceiling. Look at your outstretched fingers and hold your breath in for a moment.

Breathe out, bring your arm down, swivel over to the right, and repeat the series facing right.

Seated Sun Pose (pictured, pages 95–96)
Add the next two exercises between the Baby Pose and the Cobra Pose (pages 34–35). Bring both legs straight out in front of you and flex your toes. Sit straight, breathe out with your arms at your sides,

then breathe in as you raise your arms in a wide circle to the sides and overhead. Press your palms together, look up, visualize the sun, and stretch from the rib cage. Hold your breath in for a moment.

Breathe out as you bend forward, tucking your chin toward your chest. Grasp your ankles, bend your elbows, and pull your torso toward your legs (remember to pull by bending your arms, not by pushing with your lower back). Hold your breath out for a moment.

If you are limber enough to reach your feet (and still bend your elbows), grasp your big toes as shown on page 96 (Figure 6.39).

Release and breathe in, bringing your arms to the sides and over your head again. Stretch and look up as before. Breathe out and bring your arms back down to your sides. Repeat three times.

Bow Pose
Lie on your stomach with your forehead to the floor. Bend your knees and grasp your ankles or feet with your hands (Figure 6.31; you may have to separate your legs slightly to reach). Breathe in as you lift and

look up, pulling up on your feet so you balance on your stomach. Look up through your forehead (Figure 6.32). Visualize yourself as a bow. Hold your breath in for a moment. Breathe out and release. Repeat twice more.

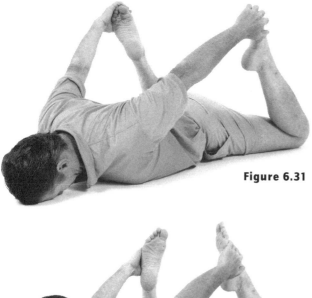

Figure 6.31

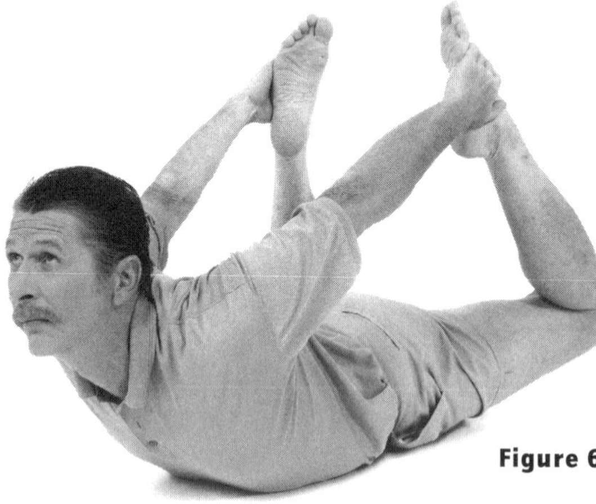

Figure 6.32

> *When I do Yoga, that's my time to relax and stretch and get a lot more limber. I've found that it helps to push me—when I almost want to give up—to that extra 20 minutes that I could have cut back and not done. With Yoga, holding postures have made my legs stronger so I can go that extra mile. When I train or do Yoga, I feel like I get into a place where I almost become this inner spirit that is able to come out in me, and I block out everything else around me.*
>
> —Aireal Evans, in-line skater

Fish Pose

Add this exercise between the Cobra Pose and the Knee Squeeze (pages 35–36). With your legs straight in front of you, lean back on first one elbow, then both. Arch your back and gently lower yourself until the top of your head rests on the floor (Figure 6.33). Place your hands flat, palms down, at your sides. Hold for a few moments, looking up through your forehead. Breathe normally.

Variation: if your knees and hips are very limber, start by sitting between your feet. Your knees should be as close together as you can manage comfortably (Figure 6.34). Proceed as in the opening pose.

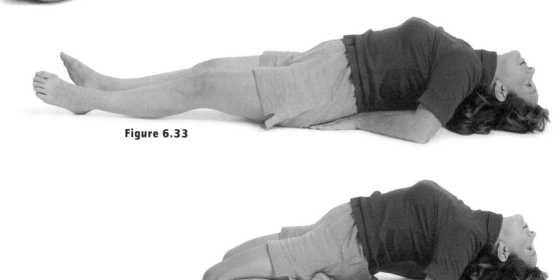

Figure 6.33

Figure 6.34

Humming Breath

Add this exercise after the Knee Squeeze (page 36). Sit up in a comfortable position, either cross-legged or sitting on your feet, or sit on the edge of a chair with your hands on your knees. Breathe in completely just as you would in the Complete Breath, described on page 20. Now breathe out with an audible *hummmm* sound, making the tone steady and loud until your breath is gone—just like the sound of a bumblebee. Let the sound vibrate in your throat, and keep pushing with your belly muscles so that the sound doesn't trail off at the end. Try to keep the sound steady. Repeat several times.

In-Line Skating

Yoga exercises can increase balance, flexibility, and strength for a more fluid motion; breathing techniques can improve stamina and focus.

In-line skating injuries are similar to those of tennis, including falls or strains from twisting, lateral, or unexpected movements. The best way to prevent these injuries is through thorough warm ups, and strengthening the abdominal muscles, back, and knees.

Modify your core routine as follows:

Complete Breath with Arm Circles (pictured, page 83)

Add this exercise before the Shoulder Roll (pages 28–29). Sit in a comfortable position as described in Chapter 2, page 20. Begin the Complete Breath exercise, but add this component: as you breathe in, raise your arms in circles to the sides and over your head. At the top, hold your breath in for just a moment as you stretch up with your fists. Then breathe out as you lower your arms in a circle back to the floor. Repeat three to five times.

Eagle Pose (pictured, page 85)

Add this exercise between the Neck Stretches and the Standing Sun Pose (pages 30–32). Stare at one spot on the wall or floor for balance. Bend your right leg slightly. Wrap your left leg over and behind the right leg (if you can't reach behind the leg, just go as far as you can). When you're steady, bend your torso and place your right elbow on your left knee. Then place your left elbow inside your right elbow, turn your hands toward each other, and clasp your fingers.

Breathe out as you bend your head so your forehead rests on your hands. Hold your breath out for a moment. Slowly breathe in, untwist, and switch sides.

Warrior Pose (pictured, page 110)

Add this exercise between the Twisting Triangle and the Cat Breath (pages 33–34). Place both hands on your right knee and lift your left leg straight in back. Bend your right knee and let your torso rest on your right thigh as you slide your hands down to support either side of your right ankle. Keep your left leg high in back. Tuck your head. Breathe out and hold your breath out for a moment. Breathe in, slowly release, and repeat on opposite side.

Variation: lace your fingers behind your back. If you can, lock your elbows, squeezing your shoulder blades together. Lift one leg as high as possible, bend your supporting leg, rest your chest on your thigh if possible, and lift your arms away from your back. Breathe out and hold for a moment. Release and switch sides.

Seated Sun Pose

Add the next three exercises between the Baby Pose and the Cobra Pose (pages 34–35). Bring both legs straight out in front of you and flex your toes. Sit straight, breathe out with your arms at your sides (Figure 6.35), then breathe in as you raise your arms in a wide circle to the sides (Figure 6.36) and overhead. Press your palms together, look up, visualize the sun, and stretch from the rib cage (Figure 6.37). Hold your breath in for a moment.

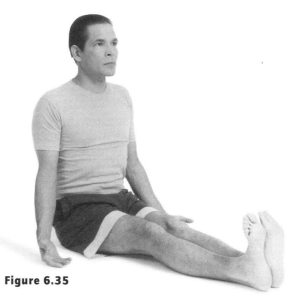

Figure 6.35

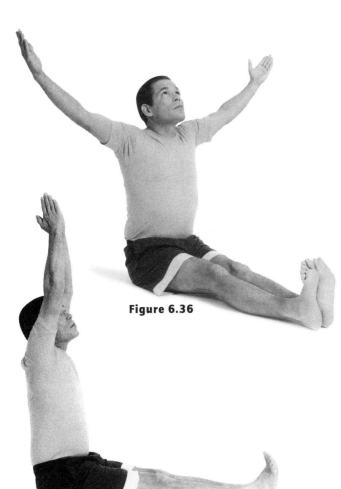

Figure 6.36

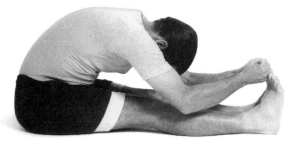

Figure 6.37

Figure 6.38

Breathe out as you bend forward, tucking your chin toward your chest. Grasp your ankles, bend your elbows, and pull your torso toward your legs (Figure 6.38; remember to pull by bending your arms, not by pushing with your lower back). Hold your breath out for a moment.

If you are limber enough to reach your feet (and still bend your elbows), grasp your big toes as shown (Figure 6.39).

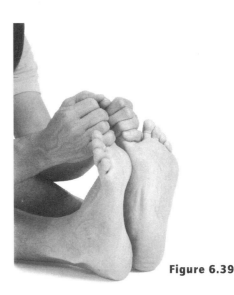

Figure 6.39

Release and breathe in, bringing your arms to the sides and over your head again. Stretch and look up as before. Breathe out and bring your arms back down to your sides. Repeat three times.

Boat Pose

Lying on your stomach, stretch your arms on the floor over your head and place your forehead on the floor (Figure 6.40). Breathe out. Breathe in as you lift your arms, legs, and head, looking up through your forehead (Figure 6.41). Hold your breath in for a moment. Breathe out and release, bringing your arms and forehead back to the floor. Repeat twice more.

Bow Pose (pictured, page 94)

Lie on your stomach with your forehead to the floor. Bend your knees and grasp your ankles or feet with your hands (you may have to separate your legs slightly to reach). Breathe in as you lift and look up, pulling up on your feet so you balance on your stomach. Look up through your forehead. Visualize yourself as a bow. Hold your breath in for a moment. Breathe out and release. Repeat twice more.

Fish Pose (pictured, page 94)

Add this exercise between the Cobra Pose and the Knee Squeeze (pages 35–36). With your legs straight in front of you, lean back on first one elbow, then both. Arch your back and gently lower yourself until the top of your head rests on the floor. Place your hands flat, palms down, at your sides. Hold for a few

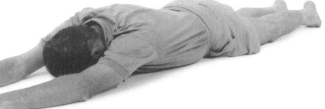

Figure 6.40

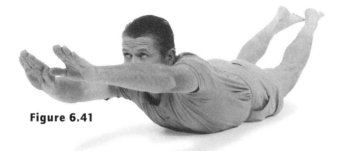

Figure 6.41

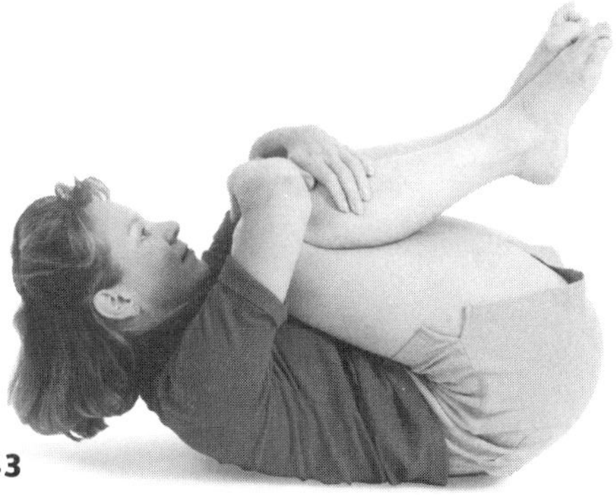

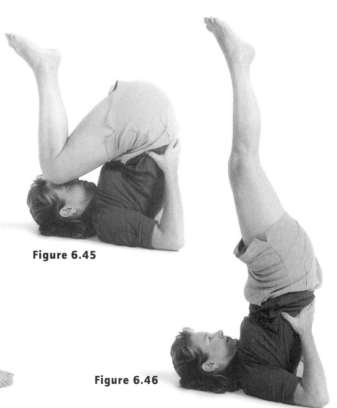

Figure 6.43

moments, looking up through your forehead. Breathe normally.

Variation: if your knees and hips are very limber, start by sitting between your feet. Your knees should be as close together as you can manage comfortably. Proceed as in the opening pose.

Shoulder Stand and Plow

Add this exercise after the Knee Squeeze (page 36). Do not do this exercise if you have back or neck problems; substitute the Easy Bridge (page 78).

In a seated position with knees bent and arms around your knees (Figure 6.42), roll back and forth a few times (Figure 6.43), then roll back onto your shoulders, immediately supporting your back with your hands (Figure 6.44) and keeping your knees bent and touching your forehead (Figure 6.45).

Slowly straighten your legs toward the ceiling and push your back straighter by using your hands (Figure 6.46). Stare at the spot between your big toes and breathe out. Hold your breath out for a moment. Breathe in and relax your breath.

Figure 6.44

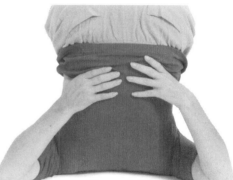

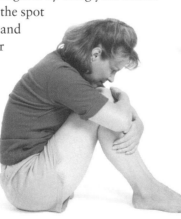

Figure 6.42

Figure 6.45

Figure 6.46

Bring your knees back to your forehead, supporting your back with your hands. Breathe in, hold a moment, then breathe out, extending your legs behind your head, carefully trying to touch your toes to the floor (Figure 6.47). Breathe naturally and hold the position for several seconds.

If you wish, try this variation: straighten your arms on the floor over your head and hold for several seconds (Figure 6.48).

Breathe in and bend your knees back to your forehead, supporting your back with your hands, then roll forward to a cross-legged position, stretching your head and arms forward (Figure 6.49). Breathe naturally as you rest for at least 10 seconds.

ENDURANCE ATHLETES GO WITH JAVA

Many athletes use caffeine to help increase performance in endurance events. If you do use this stimulant, use it sparingly, and only for performance. Daily consumption of large amounts of caffeine is not only unhealthy but also counteracts any performance boost. If you are used to drinking one or two cups of coffee daily, you won't get the enhancing effect.

Caffeine works by increasing the oxidation of fat, providing an additional fuel source to postpone the fatigue associated with glycogen depletion. About 55 percent of the population show enhanced endurance performance by drinking two to three cups of strong, fresh-brewed coffee one hour before endurance events of one hour or more in duration. The effect has been demonstrated in running, cycling, and cross-country skiing events.

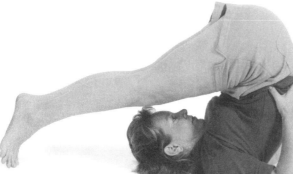

Figure 6.47

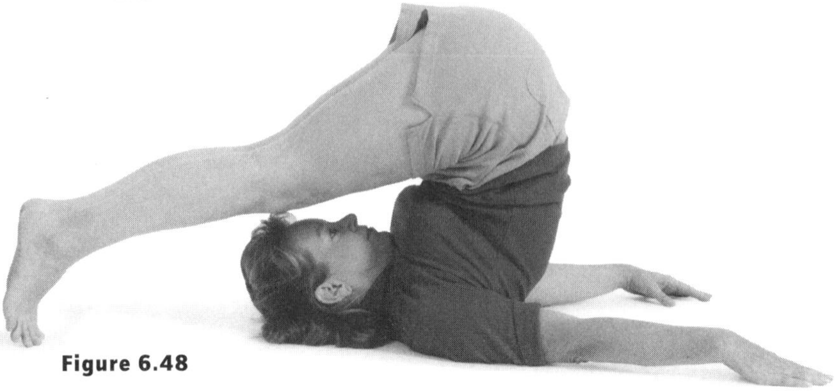

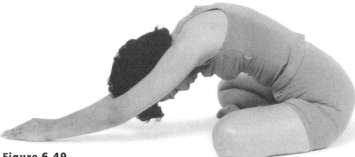

Figure 6.48

Figure 6.49

Skiing (Cross-Country)

Cross-country skiing is one of the best all-around fitness activities. Yoga keeps the spine strong and supple, providing a full range of motion in the upper body; breathing techniques can help improve stamina.

Groin and hip pulls or strains and other muscle strains are common among skiers because the arms and legs are used more actively. The best way to prevent these injuries is through all-around conditioning.

Modify your core routine as follows:

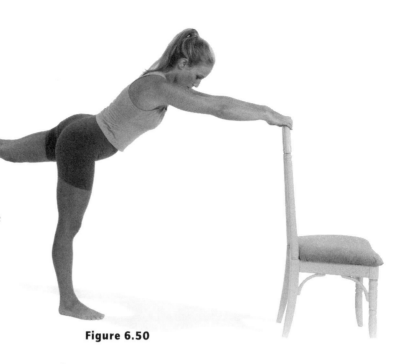

Figure 6.50

Complete Breath with Arm Circles
(pictured, page 83)

Add this exercise before the Shoulder Roll (pages 28–29). Sit in a comfortable position as described in Chapter 2, page 20. Begin the Complete Breath exercise, but add this component: as you breathe in, raise your arms in circles to the sides and over your head. At the top, hold your breath in for just a moment as you stretch up with your fists. Then breathe out as you lower your arms in a circle back to the floor. Repeat three to five times.

T Pose

Add the next two exercises between the Neck Stretches and the Standing Sun Pose (pages 30–32). When you are first learning this position, stand three to four feet from a chair or other support. Lean forward and hold on to the support with both hands. Lift your left leg in back as high as you can (Figure 6.50), ideally, parallel to the floor. Alternatively, brace yourself with both hands on the knee of your supporting leg (Figure 6.51). Keep your right (supporting) leg straight. Your torso and left leg should be in a straight line parallel to the floor. Keep your neck straight, breathe naturally, and look at a spot on the floor.

When you feel steady, release your grip on the support and place your palms together, pushing your arms out parallel to the floor (Figure 6.52). Relax your breath. Look forward at your hands. Lower

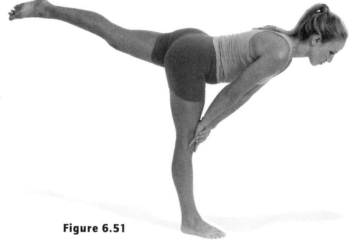

Figure 6.51

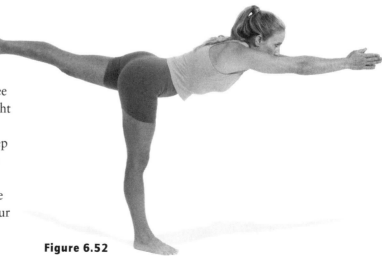

Figure 6.52

your leg and return to a standing position. Rest until your breath returns to normal. Repeat on the opposite side.

Eagle Pose (pictured, page 85)

Stare at one spot on the wall or floor for balance. Bend your right leg slightly. Wrap your left leg over and behind the right leg (if you can't reach behind the leg, just go as far as you can). When you're steady, bend your torso and place your right elbow on your left knee. Then place your left elbow inside your right elbow, turn your hands toward each other, and clasp your fingers. Breathe out as you bend your head so your forehead rests on your hands. Hold your breath out for a moment. Slowly breathe in, untwist, and switch sides.

Pigeon Pose

Add the next three exercises between the Baby Pose and the Cobra Pose (pages 34–35). From a kneeling position, slide your right leg back so you are sitting on your left foot. Your right leg should be as straight as possible, knee to the floor. Place your hands on either side of your left knee and your forehead on the floor (Figure 6.53). Breathe out completely, then breathe in as you curl up, head first, then chest, then stomach, curling back as far as you can. You can press up on your fingertips for an extra stretch (Figure 6.54). Look up toward your forehead. Hold your breath in for a moment. Breathe out and curl down, stomach first, keeping your head and eyes up until your head reaches the floor. Repeat three times.

Then push yourself up on your fists, straighten your arms, relax your back, and stare at one spot on the floor about three feet in front of you (Figure 6.55). Breathe out and hold. Breathe in as you release the position.

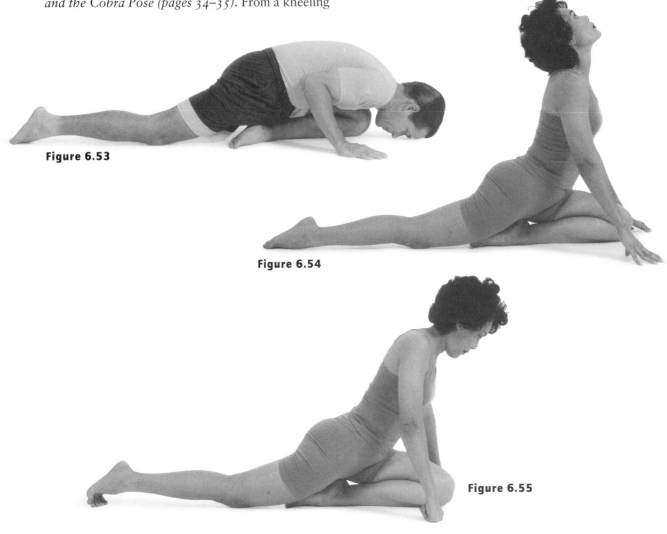

Figure 6.53

Figure 6.54

Figure 6.55

Spine Twist

Sit up with both legs bent in front of you. Bend your left knee and lay it on the floor with your left foot under your right knee (Figure 6.56). Pick up your right foot and carry it across your left knee (Figure 6.57). Pull your left foot in close to your body.

Turn toward the right and bring your left arm over your right knee. With your left elbow, press your right knee back as far as it will comfortably go (Figure 6.58), then straighten your left arm and grasp the right big toe (Figure 6.59). If you can't reach your toe, grasp your ankle (Figure 6.60) or knee instead.

Bring your right hand close in to your body, fingers pointed in, and straighten your arm. Straighten your back, breathe in looking forward, then breathe out as you twist toward the right as far as you can without straining. Look at a spot on the wall just above eye level (Figure 6.61). Hold your breath out for a moment.

Release, and repeat on the opposite side.

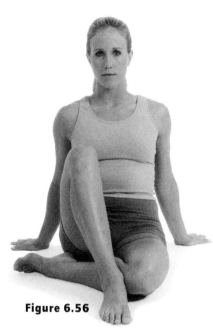

Figure 6.56

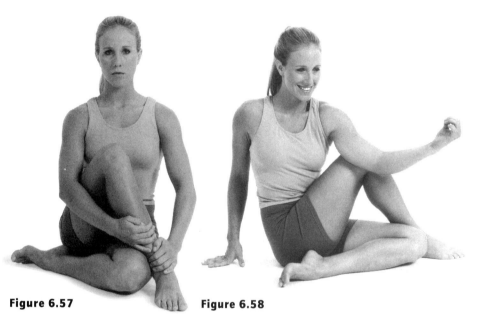

Figure 6.57

Figure 6.58

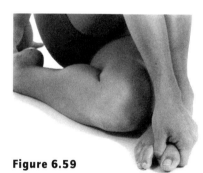

Figure 6.59

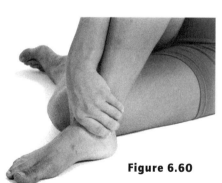

Figure 6.60

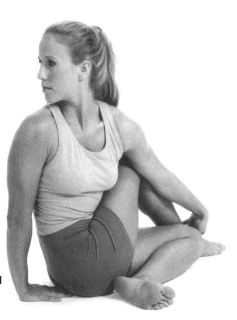

Figure 6.61

Variation: for a less strenuous pose, keep the left leg outstretched (Figure 6.62).

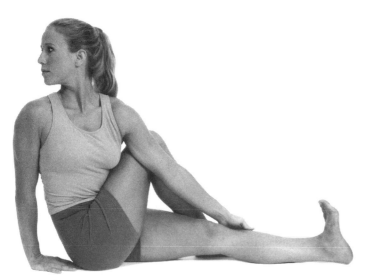

Figure 6.62

Seated Sun Pose (pictured, pages 95–96)
Bring both legs straight out in front of you and flex your toes. Sit straight, breathe out with your arms at your sides, then breathe in as you raise your arms in a wide circle to the sides and overhead. Press your palms together, look up, visualize the sun, and stretch from the rib cage. Hold your breath in for a moment.

Breathe out as you bend forward, tucking your chin toward your chest. Grasp your ankles, bend your elbows, and pull your torso toward your legs (remember to pull by bending your arms, not by pushing with your lower back). Hold your breath out for a moment.

If you are limber enough to reach your feet (and still bend your elbows), grasp your big toes as shown on page 96.

Release and breathe in, bringing your arms to the sides and over your head again. Stretch and look up as before. Breathe out and bring your arms back down to your sides. Repeat three times.

Bow Pose (pictured, page 94)
Add the next two exercises between the Cobra Pose and the Knee Squeeze (pages 35–36). Lie on your stomach with your forehead to the floor. Bend your knees and grasp your ankles or feet with your hands (you may have to separate your legs slightly to reach). Breathe in as you lift and look up, pulling up on your feet so you balance on your stomach. Look up through your forehead. Visualize yourself as a bow. Hold your breath in for a moment. Breathe out and release. Repeat twice more.

Fish Pose (pictured, page 94)
With your legs straight in front of you, lean back on first one elbow, then both. Arch your back and gently lower yourself until the top of your head rests on the floor. Place your hands flat, palms down, at your sides. Hold for a few moments, looking up through your forehead. Breathe normally.

You Don't Know How Thirsty You Really Are

Think to drink! Athletes should learn to think about drinking what is needed, rather than relying merely on thirst. Heat is a by-product of cellular energy production, and perspiration is the primary means to get rid of the excess heat. Over time, the excess water loss can lead to dehydration—a serious problem for athletes and especially for endurance athletes. For marathon runners, problems such as cramps, delirium, vomiting, overheating, and chills are all caused by dehydration. The sensation of thirst cannot keep up with need and is not a dependable indicator of adequate fluid intake. You must force yourself to drink!

Endurance events cause the loss of several quarts of water as perspiration; prolonged exercise in a hot, humid environment may result in 8 to 12 qt/day of sweat, while a marathon runner may lose in excess of 5 quarts during competition, or 6 to 10 percent of body weight.

Dark yellow urine can indicate dehydration. Force fluids until urine is copious and almost clear. Fluid loss can also be gauged and replaced by weighing before and after training or competition. Each pound of weight lost can be replaced with 16 oz (2 cups) of fluid, preferably water.

Variation: if your knees and hips are very limber, start by sitting between your feet. Your knees should be as close together as you can manage comfortably. Proceed as in the opening position.

Speed Skating

Yoga exercises will balance both sides of the body and improve flexibility, especially in the back and legs.

Speedskaters are often subject to contact injuries due to falls and muscle pulls due to improper stretching or straining. The best way to prevent these injuries is through a thorough warmup before practice that includes all-around stretching and strengthening.

Modify your core routine as follows:

Complete Breath with Arm Circles
(pictured, page 83)

Add this exercise before the Shoulder Roll (pages 28–29). Sit in a comfortable position as described in Chapter 2, page 20. Begin the Complete Breath exercise, but add this compo-

nent: as you breathe in, raise your arms in circles to the sides and over your head. At the top, hold your breath in for just a moment as you stretch up with your fists. Then breathe out as you lower your arms in a circle back to the floor. Repeat three to five times.

Leg Raises

Add the next three exercises between the Neck Stretches and the Standing Sun Pose (pages 30–32). Stand straight with both hands on your hips. (If you feel unsteady, you can hold on to a chair with your right hand.) Breathe out completely. Breathe in as you lift your right leg straight up in front as high as possible without bending your knee or straining (Figure 6.63). Hold the position and your breath for a moment. Breathe out and lower your leg. Breathe in and lift your right leg straight out to the side as far as possible without straining (Figure 6.64). Hold the position and your breath for a moment. Breathe out and lower your leg. Breathe in and lift your right leg straight out in back as far as possible without bending your knee (Figure 6.65). Hold the position and your breath for a moment. Breathe out and lower your leg. Repeat with your left leg.

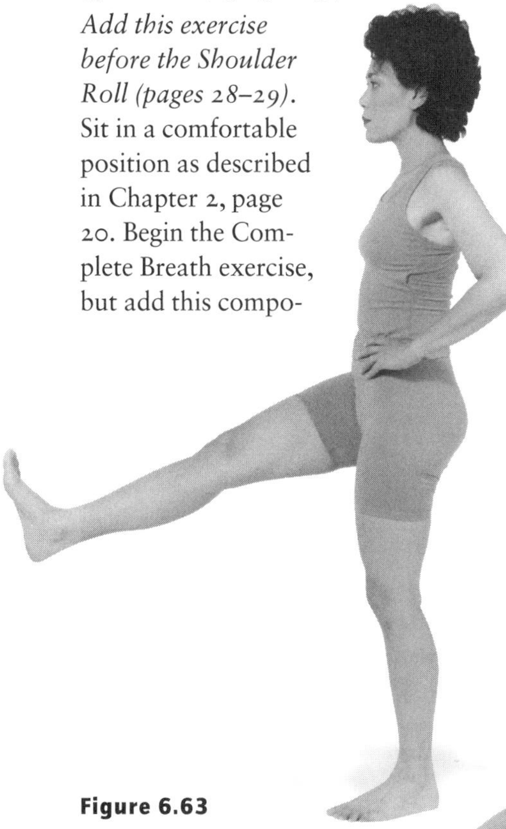

Figure 6.63

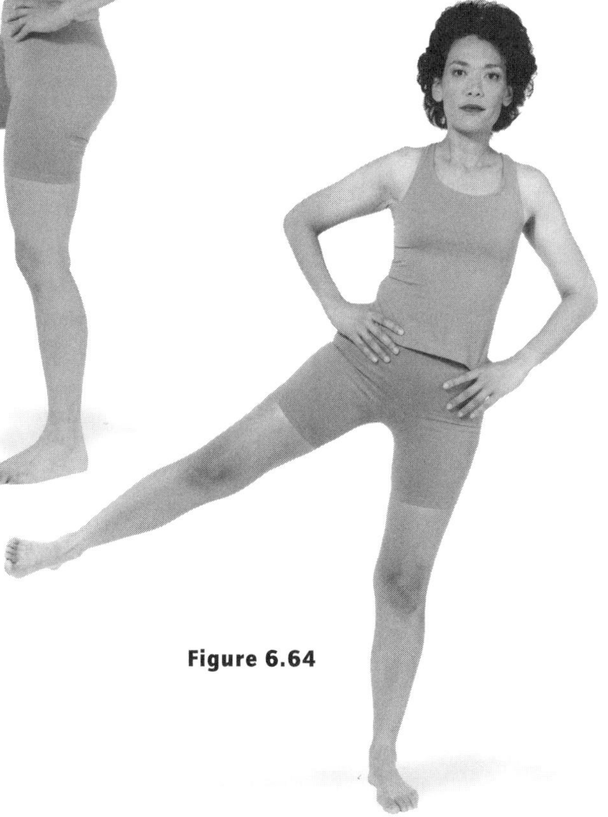

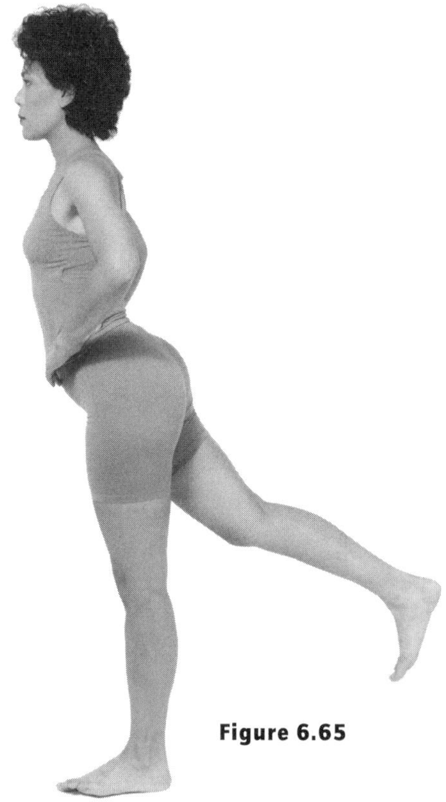

Figure 6.65

Figure 6.64

Eagle Pose (pictured, page 85)

Stare at one spot on the wall or floor for balance. Bend your right leg slightly. Wrap your left leg over and behind the right leg (if you can't reach behind the leg, just go as far as you can). When you're steady, bend your torso and place your right elbow on your left knee. Then place your left elbow inside your right elbow, turn your hands toward each other, and clasp your fingers. Breathe out as you bend your head so your forehead rests on your hands. Hold your breath out for a moment. Slowly breathe in, untwist, and switch sides.

T Pose (pictured, page 99)

When you are first learning this position, stand three to four feet from a chair or other support. Lean forward and hold on to the support with both hands. Lift your left leg in back as high as you can, ideally, parallel to the floor. Alternatively, brace yourself with both hands on the knee of your supporting leg. Keep your right (supporting) leg straight. Your torso and left leg should be in a straight line parallel to the floor. Keep your neck straight, breathe naturally, and look at a spot on the floor.

When you feel steady, release your grip on the support and place your palms together, pushing your arms out parallel to the floor. Relax your breath. Look forward at your hands. Lower your leg and return to a standing position. Rest until your breath returns to normal. Repeat on the opposite side.

Warrior Pose (pictured, page 110)

Add this exercise between the Twisting Triangle and the Cat Breath (pages 33–34). Place both hands on your right knee and lift your left leg straight in back. Bend your right knee and let your torso rest on your right thigh as you slide your hands down to support either side of your right ankle. Keep your left leg high in back. Tuck your head. Breathe out and hold your breath out for a moment. Breathe in, slowly release, and repeat on the opposite side.

Variation: lace your fingers behind your back. If you can, lock your elbows, squeezing your shoulder blades together. Lift one leg as high as possible, bend your supporting leg, rest your chest on your thigh if possible, and lift your arms away from your back. Breathe out and hold for a moment. Release and switch sides.

Lunge Series (pictured, page 90)

Add this exercise between the Cobra V-Raise and the Baby Pose (pages 34–35). With your toes pointed inward, spread your legs as far apart as you comfortably can. Breathe in as you turn completely toward the left and bend your left leg, bringing your left elbow underneath your left knee and resting on both fists. Keep your right leg straight if you can; if that position is too strenuous, rest your knee on the floor. Bend your head toward the floor as you breathe out. Hold your breath out for a moment. Breathe in and release. Repeat on the opposite side.

Breathe in as you turn back to the left. Breathe out as you rest both elbows on the floor with your left elbow inside your left knee, lower your right knee to the floor, clasp your hands, and bend your head toward your hands. Hold your breath out for a moment.

Breathe in as you push yourself up, rest your left arm on your left thigh, and straighten your right arm and your right leg. Breathe out and hold your breath out for a moment.

Breathe in and release. With your legs in the same position, breathe out as you stretch both arms out to the sides, resting your chest on your left thigh. Hold your breath out for a moment.

Bring your left hand to the floor on the inside of your left leg. Breathe in and stretch your right arm straight up toward the ceiling. Look at your outstretched fingers and hold your breath in for a moment.

Breathe out, bring your arm down, swivel over to the right, and repeat the series facing right.

Seated Sun Pose (pictured, pages 95–96)

Add the next two exercises between the Baby Pose and the Cobra Pose (pages 34–35). Bring both legs straight out in front of you and flex your toes. Sit straight, breathe out with your arms at your sides, then breathe in as you raise your arms in a wide circle to the sides and overhead. Press your palms together, look up, visualize the sun, and stretch from the rib cage. Hold your breath in for a moment.

Breathe out as you bend forward, tucking your chin toward your chest. Grasp your ankles, bend your elbows, and pull your torso toward your legs (remember to pull by bending your arms, not by pushing with your lower back). Hold your breath out for a moment.

If you are limber enough to reach your feet (and still bend your elbows), grasp your big toes as shown in Figure 6.39, page 96.

Release and breathe in, bringing your arms to the sides and over your head again. Stretch and look up as before. Breathe out and bring your arms back down to your sides. Repeat three times.

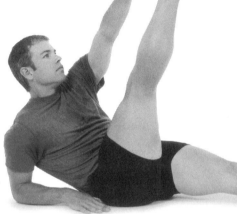

Figure 6.66

I enjoy triathlons because of the individual effort required; you only have yourself, no other assistance. The challenge comes from within. I race for myself. I'm searching for something within me; it's seldom about the guy racing beside me.

During my training sessions I first work on technique and then, as I get more comfortable, I try to empty my head of any thoughts. I try to listen to my breathing and relax my entire body. This also assists me with pain management during the long hard workouts.

In triathlons I have to search for that almost nothingness, being in the moment, because any place other than that is painful. I try to relax my body, calm my thoughts, and control my breathing so that I can get into that space—that nothingness, in-the-moment kind of space.

—Dale O'Hara, triathlete

Alternate Big Sit-Up

Lie on your back with your arms at your sides. Bring your left arm over your head on the floor and breathe out. Breathe in as you lift your left arm and right leg (opposites) and touch your toes, supporting yourself on your right elbow (Figure 6.66). Hold your breath in for a moment. Breathe out and lower. Repeat three times on each side.

Swimming

Yoga exercises can provide essential weight-bearing exercises, overall flexibility, and stronger shoulders. Breathing and meditation can improve stamina and concentration.

Swimmers often experience shoulder problems from overuse, inflammation of the rotator cuff caused by fatigue and overuse, and inflexible shoulders. The best way to prevent these injuries is to strengthen the shoulders, and through overall stretching to warm up.

Modify your core routine as follows:

Complete Breath with Arm Circles
(pictured, page 83)

Add this exercise before the Shoulder Roll (pages 28–29). Sit in a comfortable position as described in Chapter 2, page 20. Begin the Complete Breath exercise, but add this component: as you breathe in, raise your arms in circles to the sides and over your head. At the top, hold your breath in for just a moment as you stretch up with your fists. Then breathe out as you lower your arms in a circle back to the floor. Repeat three to five times.

Full Bend Variation

Add this exercise between the Neck Stretches and the Standing Sun Pose (pages 30–32). Stand with feet parallel. Clasp your hands behind your back. If you can, press your palms together (Figure 6.67). For an even greater stretch, lock your elbows so your shoulder blades are squeezed together. Breathe in and lift your arms in back as far as you can without straining. Breathe out and bend forward, tucking your chin and keeping your arms in position (Figure 6.68).

Hold your breath out for a moment. Breathe in and straighten. Repeat the exercise twice more.

hands. Raise your hips and lower your shoulders until your body is in a straight line supported on your hands and feet (Figure 6.69). Shift your weight to your right arm and breathe in as you lift your left arm straight in front of you (Figure 6.70). Focus your gaze on your outstretched hand. Hold your breath in for a moment. Breathe out and release.

Still supporting yourself on your right arm, breathe in as you bring your left arm to the side and up toward the ceiling (Figure 6.71). This will twist your body to the left as well. Look up toward your hand. Hold your breath in for a moment. Breathe out, bring your left hand down to the floor, and repeat the sequence on the opposite side. Then rest lying on your stomach.

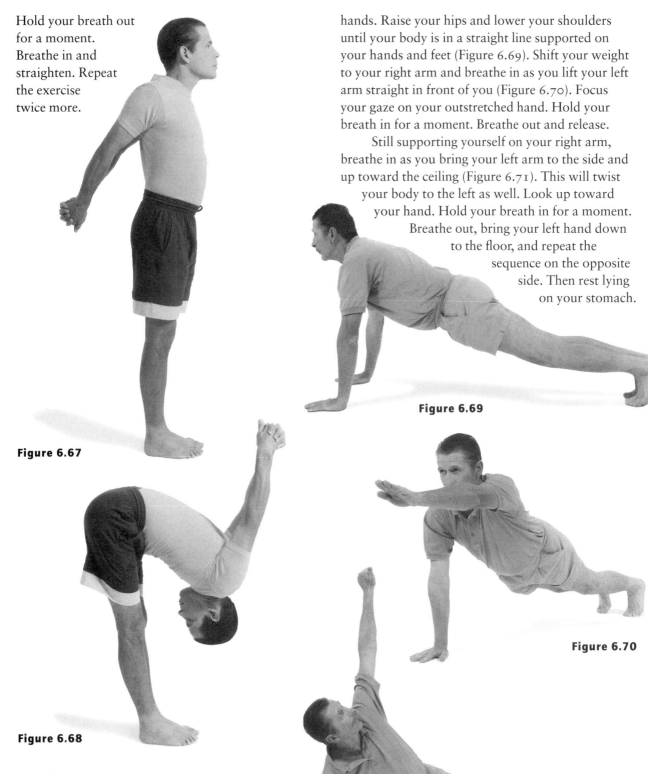

Figure 6.67

Figure 6.69

Figure 6.68

Figure 6.70

Figure 6.71

Plank Poses

Add this exercise between the Twisting Triangle and the Cat Breath (pages 33–34). From a hands-and-knees position, straighten your legs out behind you, supporting yourself on your

Arm and Leg Balance

Add the next two exercises between the Cat Breath and the Cobra V-Raise (page 34). Start on your hands and knees. Breathe out completely, then breathe in as you lift your left arm and right leg (opposites) parallel to the floor (Figure 6.72). Stare at one spot and hold your breath in for a moment. Breathe out, release, and repeat with the opposite arm and leg. Repeat three times on each side.

Variation: lift the arm and leg on the same side of the body (Figure 6.73).

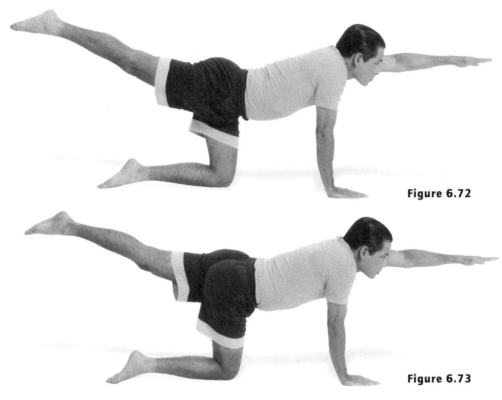

Figure 6.72

Figure 6.73

Crow Pose (pictured, page 111)

Squat on your toes, separate your knees, and place your hands on the floor between your knees about a foot apart. Bend your elbows and place the inside joint of your knees on your elbows (you'll have to lift your hips slightly). Carefully lean forward, resting your bent knees on the back of your elbows, until your feet come off the floor. Breathe out and stare at one spot on the floor. Hold your breath out for a moment. Relax and rest.

Lunge Series (pictured, page 90)

Add this exercise between the Cobra V-Raise and the Baby Pose (pages 34–35). With your toes pointed inward, spread your legs as far apart as you comfortably can. Breathe in as you turn completely toward the left and bend your left leg, bringing your left elbow underneath your left knee and resting on both fists. Keep your right leg straight if you can; if that position is too strenuous, rest your knee on the floor. Bend your head toward the floor as you breathe out. Hold your breath out for a moment. Breathe in and release. Repeat on the opposite side.

Breathe in as you turn back to the left. Breathe out as you rest both elbows on the floor with your left elbow inside your left knee, lower your right knee to the floor, clasp your hands, and bend your head toward your hands. Hold your breath out for a moment.

Breathe in as you push yourself up, rest your left arm on your left thigh, and straighten your right arm and your right leg. Breathe out and hold your breath out for a moment.

Breathe in and release. With your legs in the same position, breathe out as you stretch both arms out to the sides, resting your chest on your left thigh. Hold your breath out for a moment.

Bring your left hand to the floor on the inside of your left leg. Breathe in and stretch your right arm straight up toward the ceiling. Look at your outstretched fingers and hold your breath in for a moment.

Breathe out, bring your arm down, swivel over to the right, and repeat the series facing right.

Hero Pose Variation

Add this exercise between the Baby Pose and the Cobra Pose (pages 34–35). Sit on your heels and lift your arms overhead, placing one hand flat on the other (Figure 6.74). Breathe in deeply while rising off your heels a few inches, then begin to breathe out and slide to the left. Finish exhaling as you sit down (Figure 6.75). Try to keep your knees on the floor as you move. Now breathe in and lift up again and over to the right, breathing out as you sit down. Repeat three times to each side, alternating.

Wheel

Add this exercise between the Cobra Pose and the Knee Squeeze (pages 35–36). Lie on your back with your knees bent. Place your hands next to your head, fingers pointing toward your feet (Figure 6.76). Breathe in and push up so you are resting on your head (Figure 6.77). If you can, continue pushing up into the full position (Figure 6.78). Hold your breath in for a moment.

Breathe out and lower your body to the floor, straighten your legs, bring your arms down to your sides, and rest.

Note: if this exercise is too difficult, substitute the Easy Bridge (page 78).

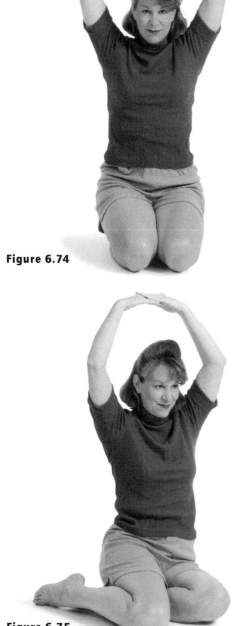

Figure 6.74

Figure 6.75

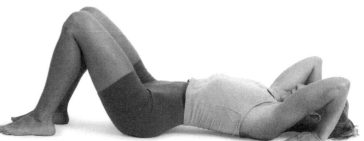

Figure 6.76

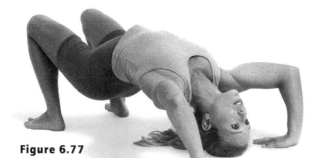

Figure 6.77

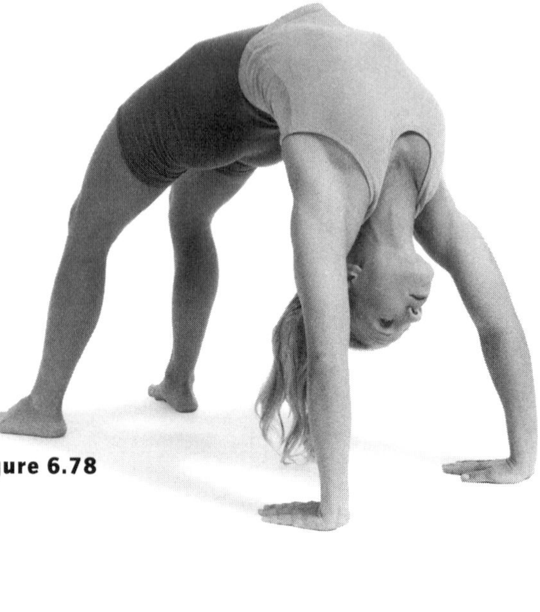

Figure 6.78

I think there's been more going on than just basketball. I always think there's a purpose to everything out there, and it's not just another job. God has a purpose for me. I think it's a calling. It's not just about coming out and picking up a paycheck and just playing basketball, and it's not just about winning the games. It's the other lessons that the boys learn. Like teamwork, like how to accept losses, how to accept wins. How to be a sportsman either way. To learn how to give a hundred percent. And learn when you're done, you're done. You leave it there. Not carry it home with you. And then to learn your limitations. Life will teach them that along the way, and it's a good lesson to learn while you're playing sports. There are some disappointments, there are some high times, there are some low times. It's all part of the big plan.

—Lemuel Andrews

Basketball

Basketball requires strong legs, back, ankles, and knee joints; agility and quick reaction time; and the capacity for team communication. Yoga exercises can help strengthen legs and joints, provide all-around flexibility training, and strengthen the lower back. Yoga breathing and meditation techniques can improve stamina and increase the intuitive communication needed for team play.

Strains and muscle pulls in the shoulder, hamstring, knee, and calf are common for basketball players, as is lower back pain, and Achilles' tendinitis. The best way to prevent these injuries is through general conditioning, including strengthening and stretching the most-used joints and muscles.

Modify your core routine as follows:

Complete Breath with Arm Circles
(pictured, page 83)
Add the next two exercises before the Shoulder Roll (pages 28–29). Sit in a comfortable position as described in Chapter 2, page 20. Begin the Complete Breath exercise, but add this component: as you breathe in, raise your arms in circles to the sides and over your head. At the top, hold your breath in for just a moment as you stretch up with your fists. Then breathe out as you lower your arms in a circle back to the floor. Repeat three to five times.

Eye Exercise
Hold a pencil (or just your thumb) out at arm's length (Figure 6.79). Focus your eyes on the tip of the pencil. Now shift your focus to an object at the far end of the room, for example a lamp or picture. Shift your focus back and forth from the pencil to the far wall a few more times. Don't strain. Close your eyes and relax.

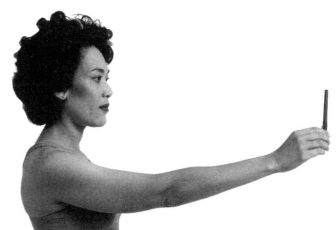

Figure 6.79

Elbow Touch
Add this exercise between the Elbow Twist and the Arm Circles (pages 29–30). Place your fingers on your shoulders, elbows out to the sides. Breathing normally, move your elbows toward each other in front (Figure 6.80), then squeeze them toward each other in back (Figure 6.81), keeping them at the same level. Repeat several times.

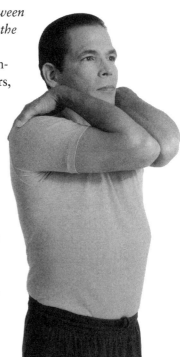

Figure 6.80

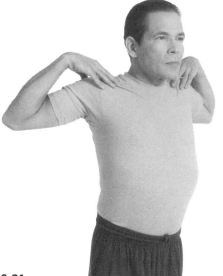

Figure 6.81

Eagle Pose (pictured, page 85)

Add this exercise between the Neck Stretches and the Standing Sun Pose (pages 30–32). Stare at one spot on the wall or floor for balance. Bend your right leg slightly. Wrap your left leg over and behind the right leg (if you can't reach behind the leg, just go as far as you can). When you're steady, bend your torso and place your right elbow on your left knee. Then place your left elbow inside your right elbow, turn your hands toward each other, and clasp your fingers. Breathe out as you bend your head so your forehead rests on your hands. Hold your breath out for a moment. Slowly breathe in, untwist, and switch sides.

Warrior Pose

Add this exercise between the Twisting Triangle and the Cat Breath (pages 33–34). Place both hands on your right knee and lift your left leg straight in back. Bend your right knee and let your torso rest on your right thigh as you slide your hands down to support either side of your right ankle (Figures 6.82 and 6.83). Keep your left leg high in back. Tuck your head. Breathe out and hold your breath out for a moment. Breathe in, slowly release, and repeat on the opposite side.

Variation: lace your fingers behind your back. If you can, lock your elbows, squeezing your shoulder blades together. Lift one leg as high as possible, bend your supporting leg, rest your chest on your thigh if possible, and lift your arms away from your back (Figure 6.84). Breathe out and hold for a moment. Release and switch sides.

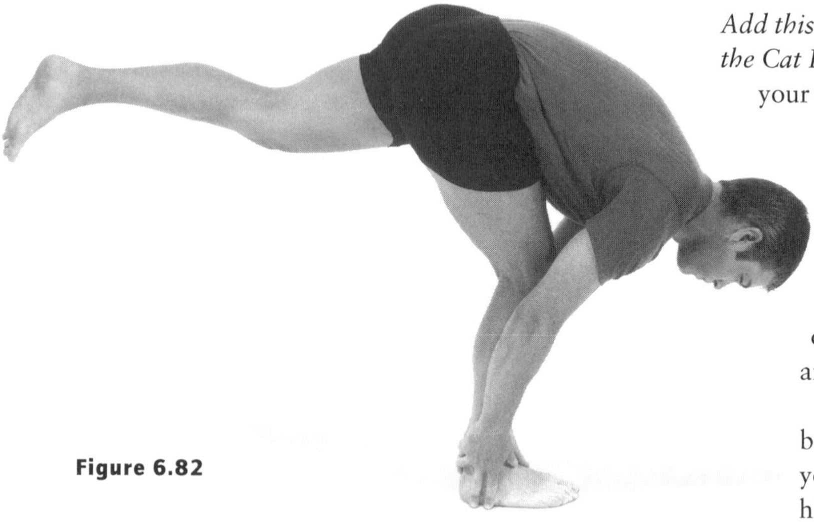

Figure 6.82

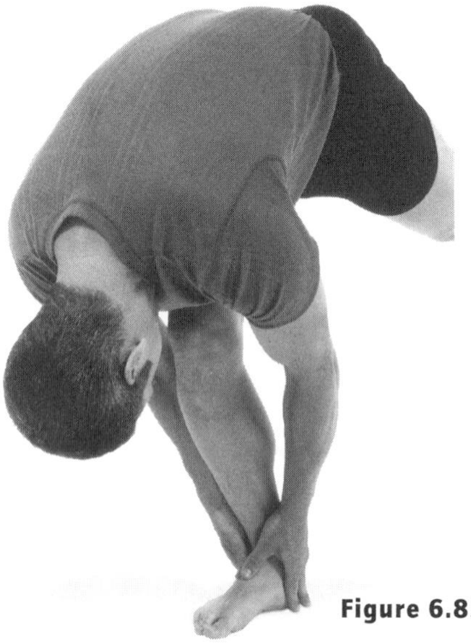

Figure 6.83

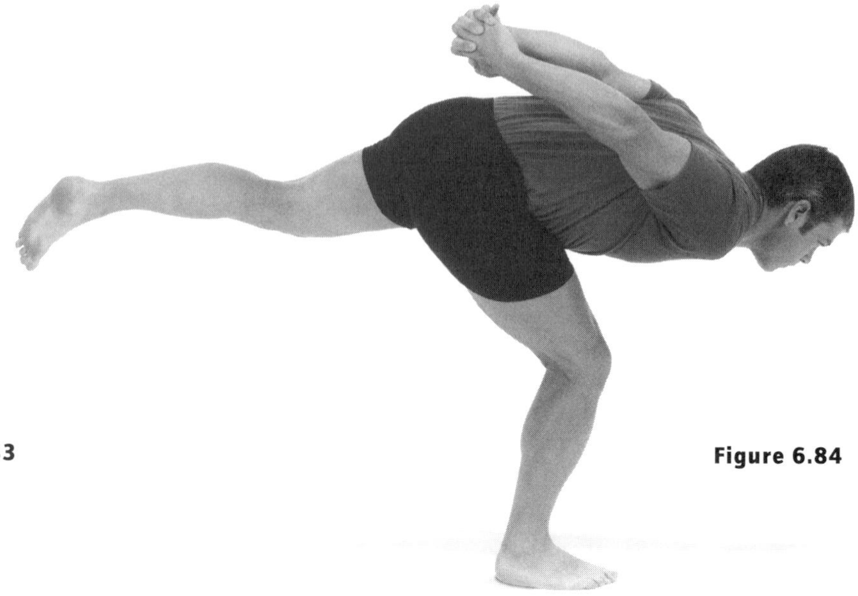

Figure 6.84

Arm and Leg Balance (pictured, page 130)

Add the next two exercises between the Cat Breath and the Cobra V-Raise (page 34). Start on your hands and knees. Breathe out completely, then breathe in as you lift your left arm and right leg (opposites) parallel to the floor. Stare at one spot and hold your breath in for a moment. Breathe out, release, and repeat with the opposite arm and leg. Repeat three times on each side.

Variation: lift the arm and leg on the same side of the body.

Crow Pose

Squat on your toes, separate your knees, and place your hands on the floor between your knees about a foot apart. Bend your elbows and place the inside joint of your knees on your elbows (Figure 6.85; you'll have to lift your hips slightly to do this). Carefully lean forward, resting your bent knees on the back of your elbows, until your feet come off the floor (Figure 6.86). Breathe out and stare at one spot on the floor. Hold your breath out for a moment. Relax and rest.

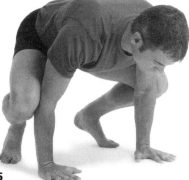

Figure 6.85

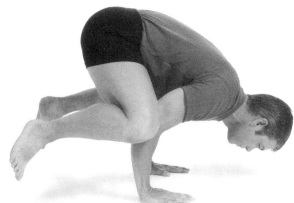

Figure 6.86

Lunge Series (pictured, page 90)

Add the next two exercises between the Cobra V-Raise and the Baby Pose (pages 34–35). With your toes pointed inward, spread your legs as far apart as you comfortably can. Breathe in as you turn completely toward the left and bend your left leg, bringing your left elbow underneath your left knee and resting on both fists. Keep your right leg straight if you can; if that position is too strenuous, rest your knee on the floor. Bend your head toward the floor as you breathe out. Hold your breath out for a moment. Breathe in and release. Repeat on the opposite side.

Breathe in as you turn back to the left. Breathe out as you rest both elbows on the floor with your left elbow inside your left knee, lower your right knee to the floor, clasp your hands, and bend your head toward your hands. Hold your breath out for a moment.

Breathe in as you push yourself up, rest your left arm on your left thigh, and straighten your right arm and your right leg. Breathe out and hold your breath out for a moment.

Breathe in and release. With your legs in the same position, breathe out as you stretch both arms out to the sides, resting your chest on your left thigh. Hold your breath out for a moment.

Bring your left hand to the floor on the inside of your left leg. Breathe in and stretch your right arm straight up toward the ceiling. Look at your outstretched fingers and hold your breath in for a moment.

Breathe out, bring your arm down, swivel over to the right, and repeat the series facing right.

Plank Pose (pictured, page 106)

Straighten your legs out behind you, supporting yourself on your hands. Raise your hips and lower your shoulders until your body is in a straight line supported on your hands and feet. Shift your weight to your right arm and breathe in as you lift your left arm straight in front of you. Focus your gaze on your outstretched hand. Hold your breath in for a moment. Breathe out and release.

Still supporting yourself on your right arm, breathe in as you bring your left arm to the side and up toward the ceiling. This will twist your body to the left as well. Look up toward your hand. Hold your breath in for a moment. Breathe out, bring your left hand down to the floor, and repeat the sequence on the opposite side. Then rest lying on your stomach.

Side Stretch

Add this exercise between the Baby Pose and the Cobra Pose (pages 34–35). Sit up in a comfortable cross-legged position. Breathe in, then breathe out as you lean to the right and stretch your left arm up over your head and toward the right, stretching the entire left side of your torso (Figure 6.87). Hold your breath out for a moment. Breathe in as you release, then repeat on the opposite side.

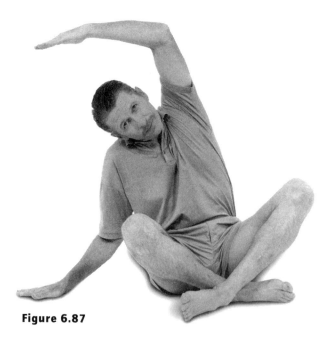

Figure 6.87

7

SPORT AS ART

Dance, Aerobics, Figure Skating, Gymnastics, and Diving

When you are watching a performance you can always tell who has the experience and past training and who is new out there. One is doing a beautiful job, but you can tell the person is working so hard to do it. The other—it just flows forth. It looks effortless. Experienced performers deliver more than just the technical part. They don't look exciting unless they have that inner drama. There's got to be something in any dance piece that has beauty in it. Because that's what gives the performer strength, a reason for being.

I think a lot of dancing depends on stamina, because most of the time you are under tremendous pressure.

—ROSEMARY SWAIN, DANCER

In ancient societies such as Greece and India, people considered the divine force of the world to be an everyday presence. They looked upon the sacrifice of athletes in training, discipline, and constant effort as an offering to the divine force of the gods. This offering consisted of intense feelings of the pain of effort, the joy of winning, and, equally important, the grief of losing. All three of these emotions held great meaning as a divine sacrifice. It was the only type of sacrifice that could be properly offered to the presence of the inner divine force that lies in humankind. The entire society appreciated these emotions because they represented gifts from the known world and its people to the fearsome power of the unknown. It was considered that human beings had the greatest ability to express these emotions, and because of this, they became the vehicle for sacrificial offering. This essential quality gave humankind importance. Humans could now communicate with the gods.

No longer inexpressive slaves in the tumultuous, unpredictable world, humankind gained a valuable bargaining tool in the loss of physical ego that accompanied the intense feeling of sports. This loss of physical ego meant that the gods gained a way to express themselves and were able to become known through the inner spiritual/emotional/power body. Loss of self provides a channel for that inner body to play, move, and speak.

Artistic sports still remain the greatest example of this phenomenon. The expression of the emotional/spiritual/power body is clearly evident when a dancer or athlete creates a truly transcendent performance. In order to present that perfect performance, artistic sport demands extraordinary courage. True, most of the movement has been carefully choreographed for discipline of form and movement; but resting on that—you might even say floating on that—is the performer. To present the performance from within, you need more than a fine-tuned, athletic body; you need one that will allow spontaneous interpretation that springs from the will of the inner being. A ballroom dancer we interviewed, Lee Ann Fergeson, said: "Performing was extremely satisfying, knowing that it was an expression of a part of myself that I couldn't express. It was a freedom."

There is an extremely fine line between the planned, classical diagram of movement and the personal interpretation that can take over without upsetting the presentation of the diagram. Crossing this line can be dangerous folly: the use of restraint is always the basis of magnificent artistic sport. The dancer, the runner, the diver—all have to forget themselves and their bodies when the expression of the inner body takes over. The physical body simply acts as a perfect support of strength while the real show of the ecstatic, emotional/spiritual/power state of the athlete stuns the audience as well as the performer with the spontaneous joy and beauty of the experience.

When artistic athletes allow this to happen, they can never be sure of the results, and so there is great need for courage. A Yogic routine of breath and meditation will supply the strong confidence needed to take the chance on loss of self; the chance to express what lies within.

The training discipline demanded by artistic endeavor is probably the most difficult in all of sports, because it requires this loss of self. Usually the training routine starts in childhood and governs every part of the young life of the athlete. The fatigue of constant training affects not only the aspirant but, usually, the whole family. Friends who have a dancer or skater in the family have said to me, "You know, we all have to adjust to the program." The sacrifice is great for everyone. The everyday difficulties of train-

After the hard work of going to class and rehearsals (and believe me, one can never rehearse enough), a performer should let go of the thinking and reacting and just feel, experience, and actually become the performance. Otherwise, the performance is only a demonstration in technique. This can be quite good, but it is never enough. The audience attends the theater entrusting and expecting the performer to guide them in an experience that will delight and entertain them. The key to this is beauty in some form. It connects the performer and the audience. The audience will always identify it and need it. The performer should always respect this. Beauty is the miracle. Beauty is magical yet real. Where there is beauty, there is joy!

—Rosemary Swain

> *If you're going to spend all this time in your life going to class, practicing, starving yourself, telling people 'I'm sorry I can't go out tonight,' not being able to be with your family because you're performing and everybody else is going to have Christmas together or whatever, then at least you owe it to yourself to know that you're doing the best thing that you can.*
>
> —Rosemary Swain

ing a child in skating, dance, gymnastics, or any artistic sport requires great support systems for the emotional balance of the child as well as for the entire family. These families all go through periods of extreme depressive behavior brought on by the never-ending pressures of the athlete's life. Because the drive for perfection in artistic sport is constant, the young athlete is also subject to periods of depression. It is easy to feel like a failure. The youngster needs a driving ambition to succeed and constant reassurance and support in the long, difficult road to superior performance.

Artistic sport can never depend totally on strength; it develops and uses strength only to express the movement of the body in a beauty that reveals the inner self. This unexpected, spontaneous movement of the body as it expresses the inner self is strongly supported by the physical strength gained in training. The ability to achieve loss of self appears when the athlete is supremely confident of his or her physical expertise. A bloom then rises from within, creating a spectacular joy that infects the audience as well as the performer.

One of the athletes we interviewed, Barbara Porter, described the experience this way: "when the ride is right, the horse and rider look like one unit. You must ride as if the horse is an extension of yourself, and vice versa. You must be able to cue him invisibly, with movements so subtle no one can see, and only he can feel. This is what experience has taught me—that within my hands and seat and legs there exists a power to communicate that comes from within. He'll know what you want without your consciously asking him. That is what makes a horse and rider great. That is what makes them one. And that is what makes the whole relationship worth all the pain and effort and the years it took to get

there. It consists of trust and an intense loyalty between person and animal. It is, very simply, magic."

The experience is difficult to maintain because the physical body comes forward to regain its control. A balanced Yogic routine, combined with care in nutrition and attention to lifestyle aspects, can help a young athlete grow and perform at the highest levels without sacrificing health and happiness.

Women in Sport

Women and girls in sports such as gymnastics, dance, and running must be particularly cautious of exhaustion and carefully manage their diet to avoid health problems that may arise in later years due to brutal disregard of the special needs of their bodies.

All women in sports must take extra care of themselves. The female body is not always the same; it is in constant change due to the menstrual cycle. Many times I have seen this fact ruthlessly ignored in athletic practice. The damage may not show itself until later years. Such problems as osteoporosis and other crippling effects can be avoided to a great extent by careful recognition that the menstrual cycle affects the whole body of female athletes in training and performance. Correct dietary management and meditation training are essential to all athletes, but especially to women.

Anemia (reduced blood hemoglobin) and menstrual irregularities are two interrelated health problems that some women athletes experience during heavy training and endurance events. Anemia is not only a health risk but will also reduce an athlete's ability to sustain a training program. Sports-related anemia is caused primarily by a diet lacking in adequate iron. The problem is compounded by increased iron loss due to training.

A delayed or absent menstrual cycle results in low estrogen, which is needed for proper bone growth in adolescents to avoid injury, and for maintenance of bone density in adults to avoid osteoporosis.

Most studies of female athletes' diets show that they do not get enough iron and calcium, putting them at risk for both anemia and stress fractures. They also typically have a very low level of body fat. Although less body fat may appear to be desirable in the athletic arena, it is dangerous in young women,

BEST FOOD SOURCES: MINERALS

Iron is found in high amounts in beef and pork and in moderate amounts in prunes, apricots, spinach, beans, tofu, blackstrap molasses, nutritional yeast, and wheat germ. All sources, however, are dwarfed by the iron content of fortified cereals. For example, Total® cereal contains 18 mg of iron, which is 100 percent of the recommended daily intake.

Zinc is much more difficult to obtain, with only beef, pork, and shellfish being good sources. Wheat germ, garbanzo beans, and lentils are the best of the rest, but in order to get the recommended 15 mg, the athlete needs to eat nearly 1¼ cups of wheat germ, for instance. A mineral supplement supplying the recommended amount of zinc seems to make good sense, especially for an athlete in heavy training or anyone who is losing zinc due to heavy sweating.

Calcium is highest in dairy foods: milk, yogurt, and cheese. Other good sources include tofu (if processed with calcium sulfate) and dark green leafy vegetables (spinach, turnip greens, kale, etc.). Unless the athlete eats at least four servings of high-calcium dairy foods daily (1 serving = 1 cup milk, 1 cup yogurt, 1 oz hard cheese), a calcium supplement should be used to replace the missing calcium. Trace minerals are difficult to evaluate and should be sufficient in the diet provided unrefined foods such as whole grains and fresh fruits and vegetables provide the majority of calories.

---

because a certain percentage of body fat is essential for critical biological functions.

Dancers and gymnasts seem to feel an urge to make the body "disappear" so that the expression of the inner emotional/spiritual/power body can be fully realized. The push is to make the body lighter and lighter so that it seems to have no weight at all. In gymnastics, form is everything; the body is almost an intrusion into the technical perfection of the movement. But it is important to remember that the constant efforts to reduce body fat in young female athletes can cause severe and long-term damage.

How Yoga Can Help

The breath and meditation exercises described in this book are especially helpful during high-stress periods. They heal the physical body as well as the emotional/spiritual/power body primarily by giving a complete rest to the system, allowing the mind to silence its conversation and criticism, and offering extra oxygen supply to the body.

Coaches and family members who are in constant involvement with athletes will find meditation exercise extremely useful for intuitive direction in support and instruction with the athletes in their care. This stops the constant barrage of conversation in teaching and guidance that sometimes becomes a harangue to athletes, who can get very bored and extremely tired of hearing the same thing every day. I suggest that athletes and their families meditate together.

Yogic philosophy teaches that words are coarse. What this means is that verbal communication—which takes a lot of effort—is less effective than the intuitive voice that speaks from within and needs no effort at all; in fact, its ability is limitless.

The Sport Routines

The exercise routines for artistic sports concentrate on balance and flexibility—both mental and physical. Techniques that build joint strength are also important. For best results, always include a few minutes of

FEMALE BALLET DANCERS

Because ballet demands light and lean dancers, ballerinas are notorious for inadequate diets, resulting in an increased risk of injury, especially to the feet, legs, and the joints of the hips, knees, and ankles. Inadequate food intake naturally limits the intake of vitamins and minerals, as well as calories, so vitamin and mineral supplementation is usually advisable. Particular attention should be paid to calcium intake to ensure 1500 mg per day from foods and supplements combined.

breathing and meditation in your daily practice session to encourage awareness and intuition.

Dance

Yoga exercises can enhance the qualities of extension, poise, balance, and stamina that make a performance truly great. Practice a varied routine of Yoga exercises, especially those that lengthen the spine. Concentrate on relaxing into each pose with your breath. Yoga breathing and meditation techniques will improve your confidence, focus, sensitivity, and awareness. The "I Love You" meditation technique, (Chapter 2, pages 24–26) can be especially helpful for dancers to build self-confidence and limit self-criticism.

Falls are the most common injury to which dancers are prone; using unhealthy measures for weight management can also weaken the body's systems, making the dancer more prone to injury through inattention (see sidebar, "Abnormal Eating Patterns," page 127). The best way to prevent these injuries is through a healthy lifestyle and a well-rounded program of Yoga exercise, breathing, and meditation.

Modify your core routine as follows:

Archer Pose

Add the next two exercises between the Standing Sun Pose and the Hip Rotation (pages 31–32). Place your right foot directly in front of the left, both pointed straight ahead. If you feel unsteady in this position, you may separate your feet slightly at first, but both should point forward. Extend your left arm straight ahead and position the hand as if you were holding a bow, with the thumb pointed up. Place your right hand on your head with fingers curled to hold the string of the bow (Figure 7.1).

Breathe in, looking forward at your thumb, then slowly and carefully breathe out and turn toward the left, keeping your left arm outstretched and following your thumb with your gaze. Twist back as far as you can and stare at your thumb (Figure 7.2). Hold your breath out for a moment.

Breathe in as you twist slowly back to face front. Relax your arms and your breath. Keeping your feet in the same position, switch the positions of your arms (right hand outstretched, left hand on your head). Stare at the thumb of your outstretched hand. Breathe in, then slowly and carefully twist back to the right this time, breathing out. Hold your

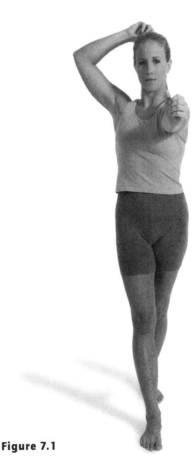

Figure 7.1

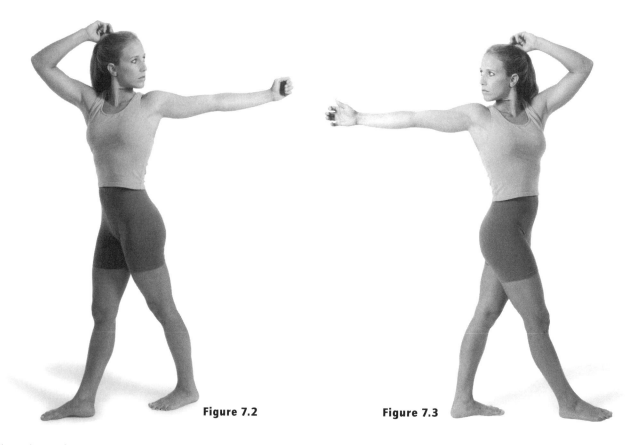

Figure 7.2   **Figure 7.3**

breath out for a moment, staring at your thumb (Figure 7.3).

Repeat the sequence with your left foot forward.

T Pose (pictured, page 124)

When you are first learning this position, stand three to four feet from a chair or other support. Lean forward and hold on to the support with both hands. Lift your left leg in back as high as you can, ideally, parallel to the floor. Alternatively, brace yourself with both hands on the knee of your supporting leg. Keep your right (supporting) leg straight. Your torso and left leg should be in a straight line parallel to the floor. Keep your neck straight, breathe naturally, and look at a spot on the floor.

When you feel steady, release your grip on the support and place your palms together, pushing your arms out parallel to the floor. Relax your breath. Look forward at your hands. Lower your leg and return to a standing position. Rest until your breath returns to normal. Repeat on the opposite side.

Lunge Series (pictured, pages 125–126)

Add this exercise between the Cobra V-Raise and the Baby Pose (pages 34–35). With your toes pointed

inward, spread your legs as far apart as you comfortably can. Breathe in as you turn completely toward the left and bend your left leg, bringing your left elbow underneath your left knee and resting on both fists. Keep your right leg straight if you can; if that position is too strenuous, rest your knee on the floor. Bend your head toward the floor as you breathe out. Hold your breath out for a moment. Breathe in and release. Repeat on the opposite side.

Breathe in as you turn back to the left. Breathe out as you rest both elbows on the floor with your left elbow inside your left knee, lower your right knee to the floor, clasp your hands, and bend your head toward your hands. Hold your breath out for a moment.

Breathe in as you push yourself up, rest your left arm on your left thigh, and straighten your right arm and your right leg. Breathe out and hold your breath out for a moment.

Breathe in and release. With your legs in the same position, breathe out as you stretch both arms out to the sides, resting your chest on your left thigh. Hold your breath out for a moment.

Bring your left hand to the floor on the inside of your left leg. Breathe in and stretch your right arm straight up toward the ceiling. Look at your outstretched fingers and hold your breath in for a moment.

Breathe out, bring your arm down, swivel over to the right, and repeat the series facing right.

Camel Pose

Add the next three exercises between the Baby Pose and the Cobra Pose (pages 34–35). From a kneeling position, separate your knees slightly, arch your back, and grasp your left heel with your left hand (Figure 7.4). Breathe normally. Do this once on each side to warm up. Then reach back and grasp both heels. Push your hips forward as far as possible without straining. Let your head gently fall back as you breathe out (Figure 7.5; unless you have a disk problem in your upper back or neck, in which case keep your head up).

Variation: if you are unable to grasp both heels at once, do the exercise once on each side in the beginning position instead.

upper body toward the floor between your knees (Figure 7.8). Your hips remain on the floor. Hold your breath out for a moment as you tuck your chin into your chest and contract your rectal muscles. Breathe in and come up again. Repeat twice more, each time bringing your head a little closer to your left knee. As your limberness increases, you will be able to lay your chest on your thigh. Repeat on the opposite side.

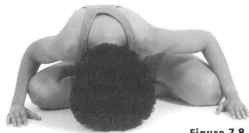

Figure 7.6

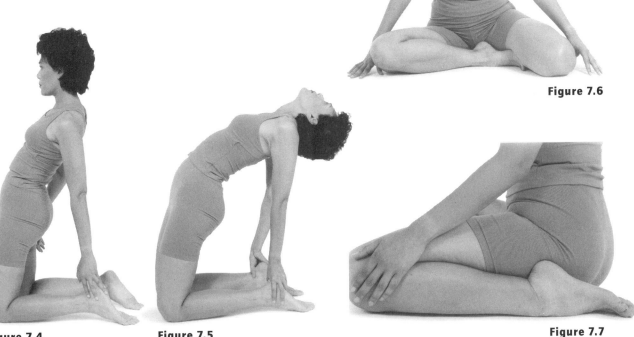

Figure 7.4 **Figure 7.5**

Figure 7.7

Hero Pose

Place your right foot on the inside of your left thigh (Figure 7.6). Curl your left foot around your left hip (Figure 7.7). Place your hands on the floor in front of your knees.

Breathe in and straighten your back. Breathe out and bend forward, stretching your head and

Figure 7.8

Diamond Pose (pictured, page 129)

Sit with the soles of your feet together, knees relaxed outward, hands clasped around your toes. Breathe in and straighten your back, then breathe out and bend forward, bringing your head toward your feet and letting your elbows fall outside your knees. Tuck your chin into your throat, contract your rectal muscles, and hold your breath out for a moment. Breathe in and release. Repeat twice more.

To limber your hips and knees, grasp your ankles instead of your feet and, when you breathe out and bend forward, press down on your thighs with your elbows.

Shoulder Stand (pictured, pages 122–123)

Add this exercise after the Knee Squeeze (page 36). Do not do this exercise if you have back or neck problems; substitute the Easy Bridge (page 78).

In a seated position with your knees bent and your arms around your knees, roll back and forth a few times, then roll back onto your shoulders, immediately supporting your back with your hands and keeping your knees bent and touching your forehead.

Slowly straighten your legs toward the ceiling and push your back straighter by using your hands. Stare at the spot between your big toes and breathe out. Hold your breath out for a moment. Breathe in and relax your breath.

Bring your knees back to your forehead, supporting your back with your hands, then roll forward into a cross-legged position, reaching your head and arms forward. Breathe naturally as you rest for at least 10 seconds.

Aerobics

Aerobic dancers, who practice a stylized form of calisthenics, will benefit from the overall static stretching of Yoga exercise as well as the calming effects of breathing and meditation techniques to counterbalance the rigors of the dance form.

The high-impact jumping and bouncing movements of aerobics are hard on the knees, ankles, and feet; muscle strains and pulls are common. The best way to prevent these injuries is through overall conditioning, warm-up with Yoga stretches and breathing techniques, and meditation to improve attention. Water aerobics are a safe alternative for those with knee or other joint problems.

Modify your core routine as follows:

Tree Pose

Add this exercise between the Standing Sun Pose and the Hip Rotation (pages 31–32). From a standing position, lift your right foot and place it on the inside of your left thigh (Figure 7.9). Relax the leg to help hold your foot in position. Bare feet will also help. If you feel unsteady, hold on to a sturdy chair. Steady yourself by gazing at one spot on the wall or floor without bending your neck. Breathe in as you raise your arms slowly over your head, straighten your arms, and place your palms together (Figure 7.10). Hold your breath in for a moment. Breathe out and bring your arms and leg

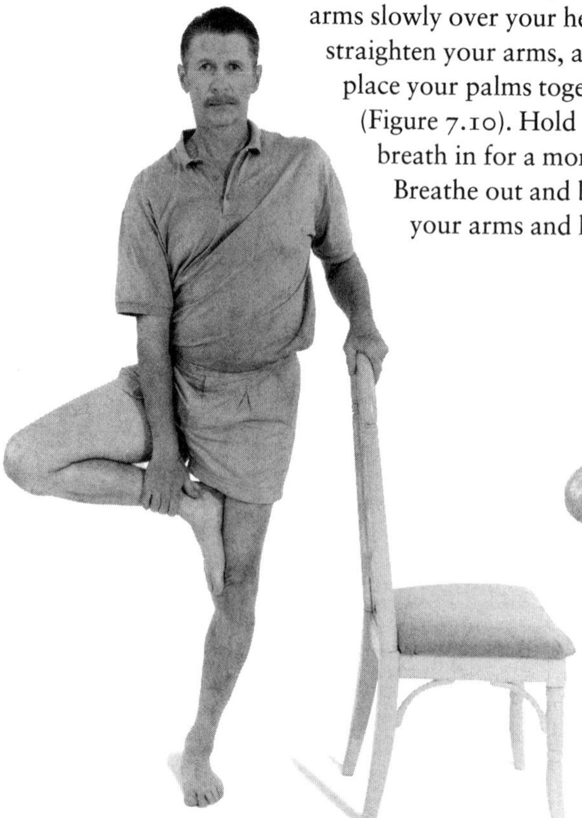

Figure 7.9

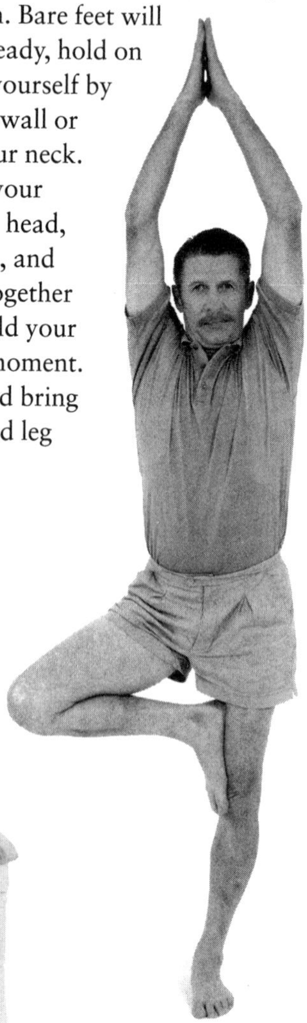

Figure 7.10

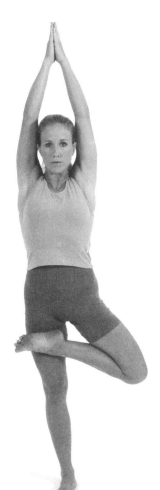

Figure 7.11

out and bend forward, press down on your thighs with your elbows.

Hero Pose (pictured, page 119)

Place your right foot on the inside of your left thigh. Curl your left foot around your left hip. Place your hands on the floor in front of your knees.

Breathe in and straighten your back. Breathe out and bend forward, stretching your head and upper body toward the floor between your knees. Your hips remain on the floor. Hold your breath out for a moment as you tuck your chin into your chest and contract your rectal muscles. Breathe in and come up again. Repeat twice more, each time bringing your head a little closer to your left knee. As your limberness increases, you will be able to lay your chest on your thigh. Repeat on the opposite side.

Big Sit Up

Add this exercise between the Cobra Pose and the Knee Squeeze (pages 35–36). Lie on your back with your arms stretched overhead (Figure 7.12). Breathe out completely. Breathe in as you lift your upper body and your legs, keeping them straight, until you touch your toes (Figure 7.13). Breathe out and relax. Repeat three times.

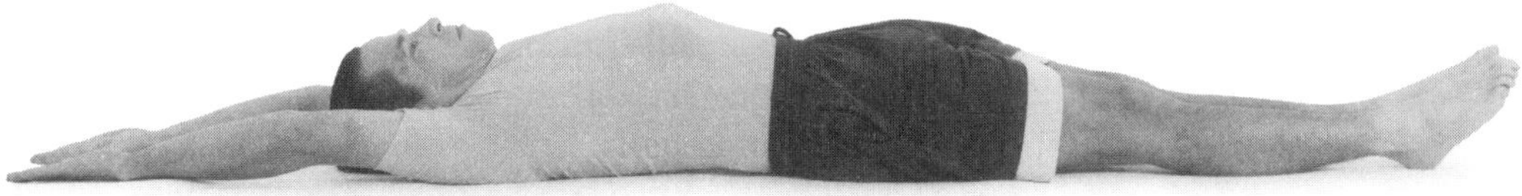

down slowly. Repeat on the opposite side.

If you are limber enough, you may place your foot on top of your thigh for this exercise (Figure 7.11).

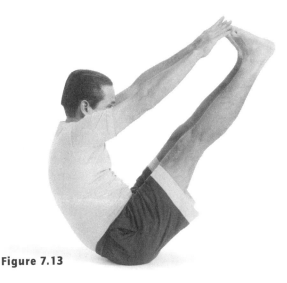

Figure 7.12

Diamond Pose (pictured, page 129)

Add the next two exercises between the Baby Pose and the Cobra Pose (pages 34–35). Sit with the soles of your feet together, knees relaxed outward, hands clasped around your toes. Breathe in and straighten your back, then breathe out and bend forward, bringing your head toward your feet and letting your elbows fall outside your knees. Tuck your chin into your throat, contract your rectal muscles, and hold your breath out for a moment. Breathe in and release. Repeat twice more.

To limber your hips and knees, grasp your ankles instead of your feet and, when you breathe

Figure 7.13

Shoulder Stand

Add this exercise after the Knee Squeeze (page 36).
Do not do this exercise if you have back or neck
problems; substitute the Easy Bridge (page 78).

In a seated position with your knees bent and
your arms around your knees (Figure 7.14), roll back
and forth a few times (Figure 7.15), then roll back
onto your shoulders, immediately supporting your
back with your hands (Figure 7.16) and keeping your
knees bent and touching your forehead (Figure 7.17).

Slowly straighten your legs toward the ceiling
and push your back straighter by using your hands
(Figure 7.18). Stare at the spot between your big toes

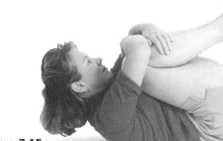

Figure 7.15

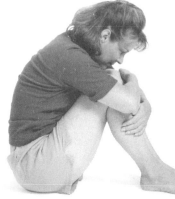

Figure 7.14

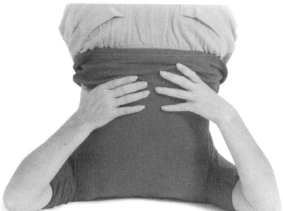

Figure 7.16

FAT IN THE DIET

The athlete's need for fat is not significantly
greater than normal. Fatty acids are used as fuel in
sustained exercise, mobilized from the body's store
of fatty tissue (adipose). Fatty tissues are replen-
ished by excess calories consumed, regardless of
food source. You don't have to eat fat to replenish
fat stores. Some fat is essential; the heart muscle
itself actually prefers linoleic acid as its energy
source, so a small amount of food rich in essential
fatty acids should be consumed daily.

Best sources for fat: olive and canola oils are the
current favorites for a healthy heart, based on the
latest results from studies of the health of Mediter-

raneans. Other good oils are sunflower, safflower,
and corn. All oils should be used in moderation; at
most only 25 percent of total calories should come
from all dietary fats. Animal fats such as greasy
meats, fatty cheeses, and butter should be severely
restricted or eliminated altogether. Most athletes
would do well to ration the following foods: butter, margarine, mayonnaise, salad dressing, ice
cream, cookies, fried chips, etc. There are now
many fat-free alternatives. Give them a try. It is vir-
tually impossible to achieve the desirable 60 percent carbohydrate sports diet when high-fat foods
are in your diet.

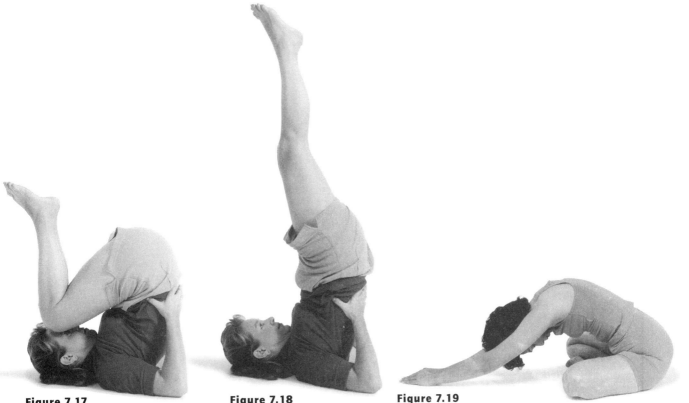

Figure 7.17   **Figure 7.18**   **Figure 7.19**

and breathe out. Hold your breath out for a moment. Breathe in and relax your breath.

Bring your knees back to your forehead, supporting your back with your hands, then roll forward into a cross-legged position, reaching your head and arms forward (Figure 7.19). Breathe naturally as you rest for at least 10 seconds.

Figure Skating

Yoga exercise, breathing, and meditation techniques provide similar benefits for skaters as for dancers. Concentrate on exercises to strengthen the back and legs and lengthen the spine, and practice breathing techniques to improve focus and self-confidence and to calm anxiety. The development of intuitive communication with the inner body will add depth and beauty to your routine.

High-speed falls can cause many injuries for skaters, particularly muscle pulls and contusions. The best way to prevent these injuries is through thorough warm-up, general strengthening and stretching, and improved focus.

Modify your core routine as follows:

Archer Pose (pictured, pages 117–118)
Add the next three exercises between the Standing Sun Pose and the Hip Rotation (pages 31–32). Place your right foot directly in front of the left, both pointed straight ahead. If you feel unsteady in this position, you may separate your feet slightly at first, but both should point forward. Extend your left arm straight ahead and position the hand as if you were holding a bow, with the thumb pointed up. Place your right hand on your head with fingers curled to hold the string of the bow.

Breathe in, looking forward at your thumb, then slowly and carefully breathe out and turn toward the left, keeping your left arm outstretched and following your thumb with your gaze. Twist back as far as you can and stare at your thumb. Hold your breath out for a moment.

Breathe in as you twist slowly back to face front. Relax your arms and your breath. Keeping your feet in the same position, switch the positions of your arms (right hand outstretched, left hand on your head). Stare at the thumb of your outstretched hand. Breathe in, then slowly and carefully twist back to the right this time, breathing out. Hold your breath out for a moment, staring at your thumb.

Repeat the sequence with your left foot forward.

T Pose

When you are first learning this position, stand three to four feet from a chair or other support. Lean forward and hold on to the support with both hands. Lift your left leg in back as high as you can, ideally, parallel to the floor (Figure 7.20). Alternatively, brace yourself with both hands on the knee of your supporting leg (Figure 7.21). Keep your right (supporting) leg straight. Your torso and left leg should be in a straight line parallel to the floor. Keep your neck straight, breathe naturally, and look at a spot on the floor.

When you feel steady, release your grip on the support and place your palms together, pushing your arms out parallel to the floor (Figure 7.22). Relax your breath. Look forward at your hands. Lower your leg and return to a standing position. Rest until your breath returns to normal. Repeat on the opposite side.

Warrior Pose

When you are strong enough, you can perform this exercise immediately after the T Pose on one side, then repeat both exercises on the opposite side.

Place both hands on your right knee and lift your left leg straight in back. Bend your right knee and let your torso rest on your right thigh as you slide your hands down to support either side of your right ankle (Figures 7.23 and 7.24). Keep your left leg high in back. Tuck your head. Breathe out and hold your breath out for a moment. Breathe in, slowly release, and repeat on the opposite side.

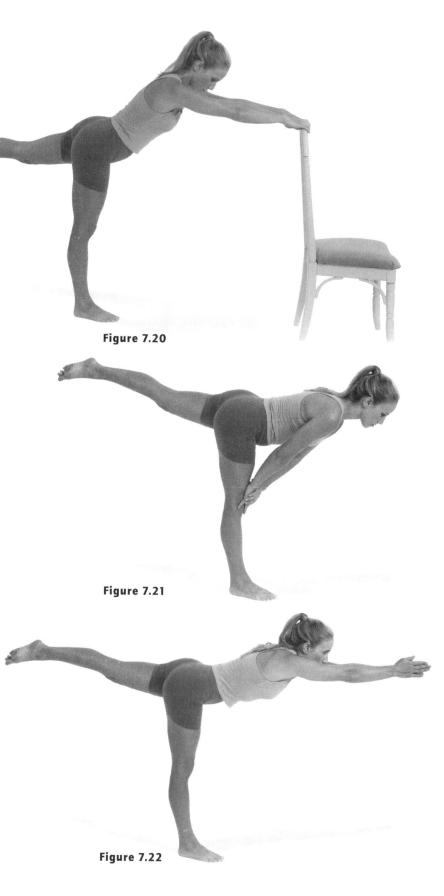

Figure 7.20

Figure 7.21

Figure 7.22

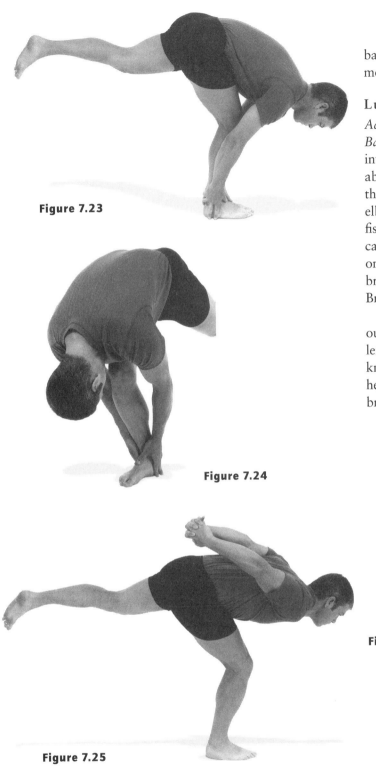

Figure 7.23

Figure 7.24

Figure 7.25

Variation: lace your fingers behind your back. If you can, lock your elbows, squeezing your shoulder blades together. Lift one leg as high as possible, bend your supporting leg, rest your chest on your thigh if possible, and lift your arms away from your

back (Figure 7.25). Breathe out and hold for a moment. Release and switch sides.

Lunge Series

Add this exercise between the Cobra V-Raise and the Baby Pose (pages 34–35). With your toes pointed inward, spread your legs as far apart as you comfortably can. Breathe in as you turn completely toward the left and bend your left leg, bringing your left elbow underneath your left knee and resting on both fists (Figure 7.26). Keep your right leg straight if you can; if that position is too strenuous, rest your knee on the floor. Bend your head toward the floor as you breathe out. Hold your breath out for a moment. Breathe in and release. Repeat on the opposite side.

Breathe in as you turn back to the left. Breathe out as you rest both elbows on the floor with your left elbow inside your left knee, lower your right knee to the floor, clasp your hands, and bend your head toward your hands (Figure 7.27). Hold your breath out for a moment.

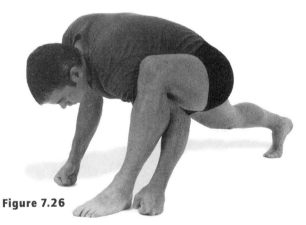

Figure 7.26

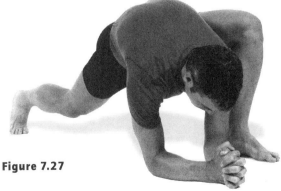

Figure 7.27

Breathe in as you push yourself up, rest your left arm on your left thigh, and straighten your right arm and your right leg (Figure 7.28). Breathe out and hold your breath out for a moment.

Breathe in and release. With your legs in the same position, breathe out as you stretch both arms out to the sides, resting your chest on your left thigh (Figure 7.29). Hold your breath out for a moment.

Bring your left hand to the floor on the inside of your left leg. Breathe in and stretch your right arm straight up toward the ceiling (Figure 7.30). Look at your outstretched fingers and hold your breath in for a moment.

Breathe out, bring your arm down, swivel over to the right, and repeat the series facing right.

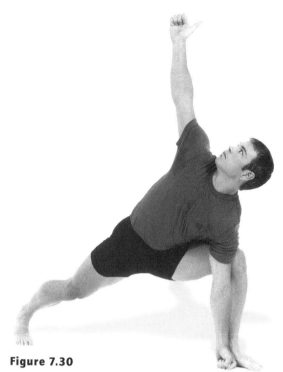

Figure 7.30

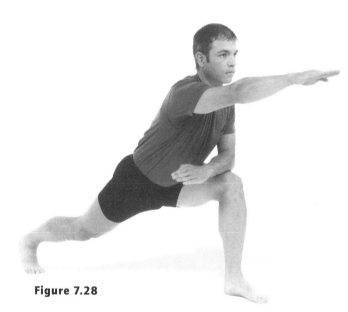

Figure 7.28

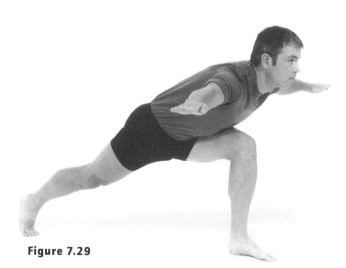

Figure 7.29

Diamond Pose (pictured, page 129)
Add this exercise between the Baby Pose and the Cobra Pose (pages 34–35). Sit with the soles of your feet together, knees relaxed outward, hands clasped around your toes. Breathe in and straighten your back, then breathe out and bend forward, bringing your head toward your feet and letting your elbows fall outside your knees. Tuck your chin into your throat, contract your rectal muscles, and hold your breath out for a moment. Breathe in and release. Repeat twice more.

To limber your hips and knees, grasp your ankles instead of your feet and, when you breathe out and bend forward, press down on your thighs with your elbows.

Shoulder Stand (pictured, pages 122–123)
Add this exercise after the Knee Squeeze (page 36). Do not do this exercise if you have back or neck problems; substitute the Easy Bridge (page 78).

In a seated position with your knees bent and your arms around your knees, roll back and forth a few times, then roll back onto your shoulders, immediately supporting your back with your hands and keeping your knees bent and touching your forehead.

Slowly straighten your legs toward the ceiling and push your back straighter by using your hands. Stare at the spot between your big toes and breathe

Abnormal Eating Patterns

Nutrition Alert: attention artistic athletes! Do you skip meals, endure 24-hour fasts, severely restrict calories, or occasionally use laxatives, diuretics, or vomiting to get rid of excess calories? Do you feel compelled to exercise away occasional overeating? Other signs of incipient trouble are an obsession with weight and an excessive fear of becoming fat. Athletes of both genders suffer a higher incidence of abnormal eating behaviors and the more serious eating disorders anorexia and bulimia, especially those in sports where their weight and shape are an issue, such as wrestling, running, dance, and gymnastics. Athletes involved in rowing and volleyball are also at risk.

Anorexia symptoms include self-induced starvation, an intense fear of becoming fat, body weight that is 15 percent or more below the normal range for one's height, and, in women, amenorrhea (the loss of a regular menstrual cycle). Bulimia, more common than anorexia, affects from 15 percent to 60 percent of all female college athletes, especially those in sports where leanness is crucial to performance, such as dancing and gymnastics. Frequent episodes of binge eating followed by prompt purging of the unwanted calories by vomiting or the use of laxatives and diuretics is common. Some may use excessive exercise as a means of getting rid of the excess calories.

Ironically, athletes harm their performance by sacrificing too much. Low calorie intake or sporadic eating results in poorer performance and endurance because of depleted glycogen stores. Low intake of protein, vitamins, and minerals leads to chronic illnesses and fatigue, makes injuries more likely, and also lengthens recovery time. Perhaps most important are the long-term health consequences for the female athlete: premature osteoporosis accompanies eating disorders and amenorrhea. (See "Women in Sports," earlier in this chapter.)

If you struggle with the vicious cycle of eating followed by compulsive exercise, or if your family and friends constantly say you look gaunt and unhealthy, you should consider seeking professional guidance and treatment.

---

out. Hold your breath out for a moment. Breathe in and relax your breath.

Bring your knees back to your forehead, supporting your back with your hands, then roll forward into a cross-legged position, reaching your head and arms forward. Breathe naturally as you rest for at least 10 seconds.

Gymnastics

The flexibility and poise needed for superior performance can be enhanced with Yoga stretching and strengthening exercises, which will lengthen the spine. Breathing exercises will help to calm precompetition anxiety, and regular meditation training will improve self-confidence and focus.

Muscle pulls and strains are common among gymnasts. The best way to prevent these injuries is by thoroughly warming up before training sessions or competition and using a full range of Yoga techniques to provide balanced flexibility and strength.

Modify your core routine as follows:

Archer Pose (pictured, pages 117–118)
Add the next three exercises between the Standing Sun Pose and the Hip Rotation (pages 31–32). Place your right foot directly in front of the left, both pointed straight ahead. If you feel unsteady in this position, you may separate your feet slightly at first, but both should point forward. Extend your left arm straight ahead and position the hand as if you were holding a bow, with the thumb pointed up. Place

your right hand on your head with fingers curled to hold the string of the bow.

Breathe in, looking forward at your thumb, then slowly and carefully breathe out and turn toward the left, keeping your left arm outstretched and following your thumb with your gaze. Twist back as far as you can and stare at your thumb. Hold your breath out for a moment.

Breathe in as you twist slowly back to face front. Relax your arms and your breath. Keeping your feet in the same position, switch the positions of your arms (right hand outstretched, left hand on your head). Stare at the thumb of your outstretched hand. Breathe in, then slowly and carefully twist back to the right this time, breathing out. Hold your breath out for a moment, staring at your left thumb.

Repeat the sequence with your left foot forward.

Dancer Pose and Extension

From a standing position, bend your left leg back and grasp your left foot with your right hand (Figure 7.31). Throughout the exercise, steady yourself by fixing your gaze on one spot on the wall in front of you. Slowly move into the completed Dancer Pose by raising your left arm straight up toward the ceiling and pulling your lifted leg up and back as far as possible without strain (Figure 7.32). Keep your right (supporting) leg straight and keep your gaze focused on one spot. Breathe in and hold your breath in for a moment.

Maintaining your gaze, slowly breathe out and lower your body into the extended position (Figure 7.33). Keep your lifted leg as far up and back as possible. Your left arm extends straight ahead. Your supporting leg remains straight. Stare at one spot for balance. Don't strain. Hold for a moment, then breathe in, come back to a standing position, and switch sides.

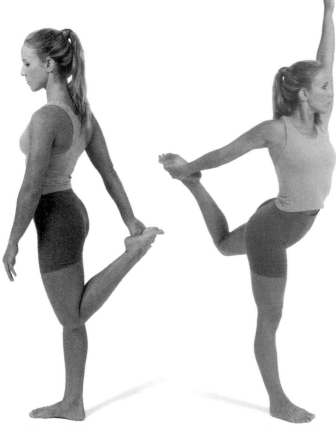

Figure 7.31   **Figure 7.32**   **Figure 7.33**

T Pose (pictured, page 124)

When you are first learning this position, stand three to four feet from a chair or other support. Lean forward and hold on to the support with both hands. Lift your left leg in back as high as you can, ideally, parallel to the floor. Alternatively, brace yourself with both hands on the knee of your supporting leg. Keep your right (supporting) leg straight. Your torso and left leg should be in a straight line parallel to the floor. Keep your neck straight, breathe naturally, and look at a spot on the floor.

When you feel steady, release your grip on the support and place your palms together, pushing your arms out parallel to the floor. Relax your breath. Look forward at your hands. Lower your leg and return to a standing position. Rest until your breath returns to normal. Repeat on the opposite side.

Lion Pose

Add the next two poses between the Baby Pose and the Cobra Pose (pages 34–35). Sit on your feet, or cross-legged. Spread your fingers apart like a lion's paws and grip your knees. Lean forward slightly and take a deep breath through your nose. Open your eyes wide, raise your eyebrows, stick out your tongue, and roar fiercely (Figure 7.34). Visualize and try to look like a roaring lion.

Diamond Pose

Sit with the soles of your feet together, knees relaxed outward, hands clasped around your toes (Figure 7.35). Breathe in and straighten your back, then breathe out and bend forward, bringing your head toward your feet and letting your elbows fall outside your knees (Figure 7.36). Tuck your chin into your throat, contract your rectal muscles, and hold your breath out for a moment. Breathe in and release. Repeat twice more.

To limber your hips and knees, grasp your ankles instead of your feet and, when you breathe out and bend forward, press down on your thighs with your elbows (Figure 7.37).

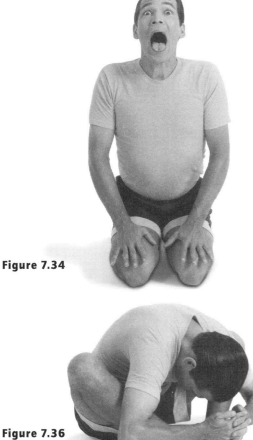

Figure 7.34

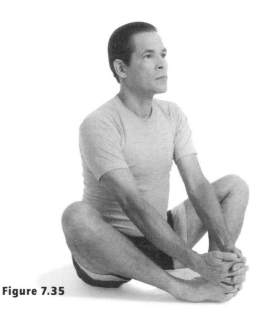

Figure 7.35

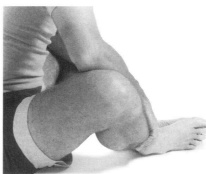

Figure 7.36

Figure 7.37

LOSING IT

Athletes who need to lose weight should avoid high-protein, low-carbohydrate diets; you won't have the energy to train or compete. Instead, be ruthless about cutting fats. Live on starches such as whole grains, fruits, and vegetables, with low-fat protein sources such as fat-free dairy products. Also, eat more of your food early in the day, so you won't go crazy with snacks at night.

Diving

Diving originated from early gymnasts, who sometimes practiced their moves over water; most dives have counterparts in gymnastic movements. Recommendations for Yoga techniques are similar to those for gymnasts: general flexibility and strengthening exercises, breathing techniques to calm anxiety and improve focus, and meditation training to increase self-confidence and intuition. Fantasy can be used to practice form.

Miscalculated movements while diving can sometimes cause injury from hitting the water in the wrong way or even striking the board or the pool bottom. The best way to prevent these injuries is through thorough warm-up and extra attention to self-esteem needs when fatigued.

Modify your core routine as follows:

Tree Pose (pictured, pages 120–121)

Add this exercise between the Standing Sun Pose and the Hip Rotation (pages 31–32). From a standing position, lift your right foot and place it on the inside of your left thigh. Relax the leg to help hold your foot in position. Bare feet will also help. If you feel unsteady, hold on to a sturdy chair. Steady yourself by gazing at one spot on the wall or floor without bending your neck. Breathe in as you raise your arms slowly over your head, straighten your arms, and place your palms together. Hold your breath in for a moment. Breathe out and bring your arms and leg down slowly. Repeat on the opposite side.

If you are limber enough, you may place your foot on top of your thigh for this exercise.

Arm and Leg Balance

Add the next two exercises between the Cat Breath and the Cobra V-Raise (page 34). Start on your hands and knees. Breathe out completely, then breathe in as you lift your left arm and right leg (opposites) parallel to the floor (Figure 7.38). Stare at one spot and hold your breath in for a moment. Breathe out, release, and repeat with the opposite arm and leg. Repeat three times on each side.

Variation: lift the arm and leg on the same side of the body (Figure 7.39).

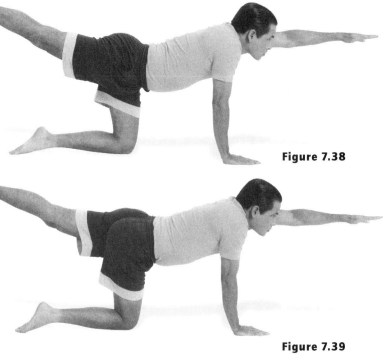

Figure 7.38

Figure 7.39

Bow Variation

Start on your hands and knees. Reach back with your left hand and grasp your right foot. Stare at one spot on the wall or floor for balance as you breathe in and lift your foot up and away from your body as far as possible (Figure 7.40). Hold your breath in for a moment. Breathe out, release slowly, and switch sides. Repeat three times on each side.

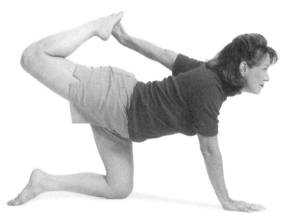

Figure 7.40

Side Stretch

Add the next two exercises between the Baby Pose and the Cobra Pose (pages 34–35). Sit up in a comfortable cross-legged position. Breathe in, then breathe out as you lean to the right and stretch your left arm up over your head and toward the right, stretching the entire left side of your torso (Figure 7.41). Hold your breath out for a moment. Breathe in as you release, then repeat on the opposite side.

Diamond Pose (pictured, page 129)

Sit with the soles of your feet together, knees relaxed outward, hands clasped around your toes. Breathe in and straighten your back, then breathe out and bend forward, bringing your head toward your feet and letting your elbows fall outside your knees. Tuck your chin into your throat, contract your rectal muscles, and hold your

breath out for moment. Breathe in and release. Repeat twice more.

To limber your hips and knees, grasp your ankles instead of your feet and, when you breathe out and bend forward, press down on your thighs with your elbows.

Shoulder Stand and Plow (shoulder stand pictured, pages 122–123)

Add the next two exercises after the Knee Squeeze (page 36). Do not do this exercise if you have back or neck problems; substitute the Easy Bridge (page 78).

In a seated position with knees bent and arms around your knees, roll back and forth a few times, then roll back onto your shoulders, immediately supporting your back with your hands and keeping your knees bent and touching your forehead.

Slowly straighten your legs toward the ceiling and push your back straighter by using your hands. Stare at the spot between your big toes and breathe out. Hold your breath out for a moment. Breathe in and relax your breath.

Bring your knees back to your forehead, supporting your back with your hands. Breathe in, hold a moment, then breathe out, extending your legs behind your head, carefully trying to touch your toes to the floor (Figure 7.42). Breathe naturally and hold the position for several seconds.

If you wish, try this variation: straighten your arms on the floor over your head and hold for several seconds (Figure 7.43).

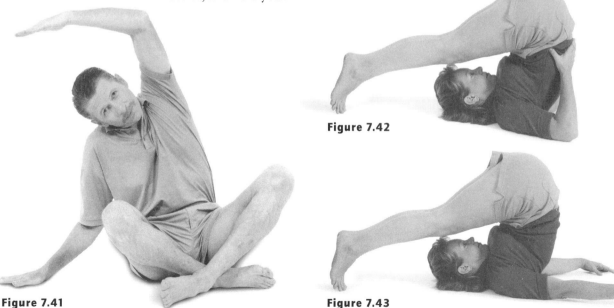

Figure 7.41

Figure 7.42

Figure 7.43

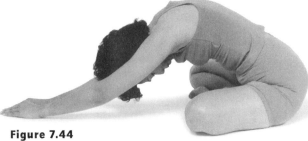

Figure 7.44

Breathe in and bend your knees back to your forehead, supporting your back with your hands, then roll forward to a cross-legged position, stretching your head and arms forward (Figure 7.44). Breathe naturally as you rest for at least ten seconds.

Wheel

Lie on your back with your knees bent. Place your hands next to your head, fingers pointing toward your feet (Figure 7.45). Breathe in and push up so you are resting on your head (Figure 7.46). If you can, continue pushing up into the full position (Figure 7.47). Hold your breath in for a moment.

Breathe out and lower your body to the floor, straighten your legs, bring your arms down to your sides, and rest.

Note: if this exercise is too difficult, substitute the Easy Bridge (page 78).

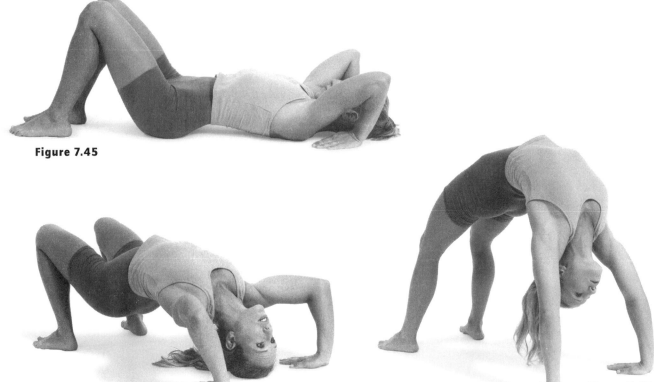

Figure 7.45

Figure 7.46

Figure 7.47

8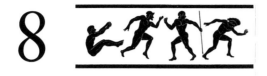

STRENGTH AND BALANCE SPORTS

Wrestling, Weight Training, Martial Arts, Surfing and Sailboarding, Downhill Skiing, and Sailing

Strength training brings on huge emotional changes because you feel so much better about yourself. You lift out of a depression state. Plus you look different. You feel different, you look different, you look better. People compliment you. It increases your morale.

—TIM WATNEM

As a player in baseball, football, and basketball, I remember times, stepping on the court, when it had nothing to do with me, I just knew that every shot I put up was going in that day. Or that I was going to have a good day on the field baseball-wise, or that I was just unstoppable on the football field. I don't know what happens. If anyone could bottle that and sell it, it would be great! But there are those moments where everything works. And mentally and physically you've done what you should have done. You're prepared. I don't think you have those moments as an unprepared player. You're in good shape, you're in good condition. If you haven't

done the preparation, I don't think you ever have those moments. I think you play to a place of consistency because of what you've done before the game. And then all of a sudden one game all of it blossoms for you. And yeah, the basket looks like Michael Jordan says, huge, like a big bucket, and you're just throwing it up there and no matter where you throw it, it's going in. I've had one or two times that happened. It's pretty euphoric.

You feel real good about yourself and your confidence level is really up there. And it's not that you're not very confident at any other time you step on the court, but you're a whole lot more confident than you have ever been. Of course you feel good about yourself. And you could take it the wrong way—start thinking that you're greater than you are. But experience teaches you after a while that you'll have one or two of those and you'll settle down after the game is over and say no big deal.

—LEMUEL ANDREWS

Personal strength, which lies in the inner body, is a great support for those practicing sport of any kind. You do not always need a perfect body to display the beauty of strength; wheelchair athletes, for instance, develop great strength in their upper body that helps them succeed despite other physical limitations.

Many sports allow a brief rest between movements. In tennis, for example, one person does not always serve; the serve passes back and forth between the opponents. This permits a small change of action in the participants' involvement, which allows a redistribution of effort and intensity that gives the body a chance to adjust.

This is not true for most of the sports covered in this chapter, however. Wrestling, martial arts, surfing, and skiing, for instance, require near perfection in physical strength because the whole body is needed for a brief spurt of intense activity during which there is no rest. (This extreme energy requirement is described as oxidative energy. The athlete must prepare for it. For a complete description of the four types of energy required by athletes, see page 11.)

These sports demand the highest performance of the body from start to finish with maximum exertion. The athlete has to prepare for an effort that requires 100 percent strength without a partner to depend upon and no chance to rest or regroup. The situation can be compared to the finish of a horse race, where all systems are on full performance for the entire time of competition. Lemuel Andrews, a coach we interviewed, expressed that push:

> Basketball is very demanding. We run and we press all the time. So I tell them, "Mentally you have to be prepared to play through the times that you are tired. You are going to be weary. And you have to play through that because the other guy is tired too. He's just as tired, and you should be in better shape because of the conditioning we've done. So when he droops down and looks like he can't take another step, I want you to walk tall. And psychologically make it."

This huge expectation of body performance rests heavily on the emotional balance and strength of the inner body of the athlete as well as that of the outer physical body. Many times you will hear a coach say, "Put your heart into it" or "Give it all you've got." The very use of the phrase "Put your heart into it" implies that the heart of the athlete lies somewhere other than the physical body. But we all know that it doesn't, so what do these phrases refer to? The implication is that the athlete has a secret power supply to call upon. Coaches know that athletes can call upon physical super-strength by centering their thought toward the inner emotional/spiritual/power body. A channel opens for that extraordinary strength to join with the outer physical body, resulting in performance success. Yoga training serves to make a bridge to that supply of emotional power strength.

I have noticed that athletes who enjoy wrestling and weight lifting are not talkative people. They are never described as loquacious and would readily agree with the old proverb "Great talkers are like leaky pitchers; everything runs out of them." The classical wrestlers I have known seem to have an instinctual knowledge of loss and are careful to guard themselves from it even in conversation. Every movement calls on a huge concentrated support from deep within the body; this remembrance leads to a

---

From what I understand, the focus for the concentration required for Yoga is very similar to that required for wrestling. A match lasts only six minutes, but the intensity is so great, so much is happening. You have to be so aware of not only your own body but your opponent's body without being able to see it, because you're in such close proximity. You have to be able to intuit it. And that requires, I think, probably a similar type of concentration. You have to be very into what you are doing. You're very much right there in the center. It's a completely different experience when you are "in the zone." When it happens to me, I just naturally slip into it, but I know I'm slipping into it. Time slows down.

— Mike Colgrove, wrestler

I see a real continuity there between what goes on in my mind when I wrestle and what happens in this prayer/meditation group that I'm in. It's very different, but there's definitely continuity, and I find that they help one another. Both things work different parts of that part of myself. They help each other because they are related. When I was in college I was a musician. I remember thinking that going to my flute performance lessons and thinking a completely different way actually helped me do my physics problem sets. The two subjects had nothing to do with each other but yet, because they gave me the opportunity to use both sides of the brain, on the whole it made both things better. Exercising those different capacities actually helped each one.

—Nelson Gonzalez, wrestler

this hidden source of strength can be available to you on call; in fact, it has always been part of your performance. The emergence of this extra strength can become predictable with practice.

The ecstatic joy of skiing is for the most part enjoyed by the individual skier. There are, of course, times when spectators can enjoy the "thrill of victory and the agony of defeat," but, for the most part, skiing is done for the fun of it. When the physical body is flexible and strong, the experience of flying down a mountainside gives the wonderful feeling of loss of self: "I am not tied to the earth. I can fly!" This feeling is supported by a physical body that can take a fall without being destroyed. Just as important is the ability to maintain consciousness in two distinct areas: the wild flying ride of the skis and the remembrance of the need for protection of the physical body. This takes balance training for the body and the mind. Regular practice of asans and meditation will give an athlete the extra quality of mental balance that is needed to become a star athlete.

natural, constant introspection. This inward direction, a natural aspect of classical wrestling, can be enhanced greatly by the practice of breathing and meditation techniques. I want to clarify, too, that this inward quality disappears when wrestlers shift from classical wrestling to the arena of show business spectacle, where talkativeness is expected and exploited.

Most athletes really never know when the extraordinary super-strength of the inner emotional/spiritual/power body will come forward in competition. It is usually a rare, remarkable experience. The addition of breathing and meditation exercises to each training workout and before competition will provide a clear channel for the super support of the inner body to flow easily. With practice, the flow becomes automatic when the physical calls for it. This means that you are not alone in what is sometimes called a lonely sport; you have called in your own troops, and enormous strength is now at your disposal—strength that does not show in the ordinary practice of physical strength training and yet is always there. Yogic techniques added to your everyday training workouts will show you that

I love skiing because of the freedom of it and the sense of exhilaration that permeates every aspect of it: moving fast, going down the hills. The most thrilling part, though, is getting enough competence in what you are doing so that something else comes in and the fear subsides and you just go. You let the skis run, and there is a natural movement where you are shushing down a mountain and the turns are automatic. You're not thinking "I've got to do this, I've got to do that." It just becomes an automatic sense, like floating. Something just takes over where you're not there. Your skis and you become one. It seems to be all feeling; your mind is not in the minutiae of what to do. You're so focused in the moment that your mind doesn't go anywhere else. Fear doesn't enter into it because you're in the moment exactly.

—Elizabeth Walton, skier

> *Skiing can be exciting, challenging, and fun. It's challenging because, depending on where you're going, you really are concentrating. You're not thinking about what the weather is like, or what's happening at home. You're a hundred percent focused when you're going down a challenging slope. And that's where your energy is. That's where your focus is. It's everything. It's just right there in the moment and that's fun.*
>
> —Krista Benz, skier

> *You want strength in the stomach because usually that part of the body is fairly weak in most people. When you are practicing sparring, you want to be able to take some blows to the stomach. And so you do a lot of crunches, sit ups. Asans such as the Big Sit-Up would really help. That whole series is great for strengthening the abdominals.*
>
> —Steve Honeyager,
> martial arts practitioner

> *You are fighting this complete physical exhaustion. There is definitely a battle of wills there. You are forcing your body to push itself as far as it possibly can in order to win the match. I don't necessarily have any really strong emotions or inclinations toward my opponent. To me it's just methodically doing the moves that I've been trained to do and countering what he's doing to me in order for me to achieve my goal.*
>
> —Michael Colgrove

Martial arts practitioners can also benefit from the regular use of meditation and breathing before practice and performance. The strong concentration that develops when you make Yogic breathing and meditation part of your daily discipline allows the sudden burst of energy that takes your opponent off guard and carries through with the strength of movement that you need to complete the attack. Extreme concentration allows you to be drawn back into the depth of yourself. A great quietness lies there, and extra strength easily arises from that state. What the opponent does is not important. You can be a total machine of concentrated strength. Nothing else can distract you from your purpose. You can intuitively know your opponent's next move.

Serious surfers and sailboarders become addicted to their sport. You feel that you have joined with the power of the world of water. A unique state of consciousness takes over when this happens that allows you to feel ecstatically free. Take special dietary care to avoid dehydration and sun damage to the skin and especially the eyes, and develop flexibility and intuition to help you avoid injury. Regular practice of asans and meditation are the best way to supply these qualities.

The sport of sailing is totally dependent upon intuition. The ability to feel the boat in the water and to judge the wind and its vagaries, and the need for overall awareness depend solely on the ability of the athlete to move away from physical body consciousness and rest on the mystical emotional/spiritual/power body within. Most of the sailors I have known over the years constantly feel the need to reach mystical depth in themselves. They enjoy this feeling so much that they try to reach it even when they are not sailing. The problem is that the most common way they know how to do it is with alcohol. This eventually becomes a detriment to their sport. Strength and health suffer.

The serious sailors I have known all also have a strong tendency to introversion. This definitely implies that the natural tendency of a serious sailing aspirant is to search for the intuitive experience of the inner body. This attribute can cause imbalance in the sailor's life because it sometimes denies the importance of normal physical life. People who sail often suffer from devastating personal relationships due to this phenomenon. If you love to sail, you need balance in your emotional body as well as in your physical body. Regular practice of Yogic techniques can help bring this balance about. Meditation practice especially will enable you to converse about feelings that are troublesome to explain. You can achieve a comfortable quality in communication that

FOOD MYTHS

Myth # 1: drinking water during competition causes cramps.

Appropriate beverages before, during, and after exercise can significantly aid performance. For nonendurance activities, cool water in volumes up to 20 oz best fits the body's needs (the addition of flavoring, carbohydrate, and electrolytes simply makes the drink more palatable). For endurance athletes (events longer than 90 minutes), small frequent doses (4–6 oz every 15 minutes) of water with light solutions (4–8 percent) of carbohydrates from sugar, glucose, glucose polymer, etc., and small quantities of sodium (to speed up absorption) are needed. Such a mild solution rapidly leaves the stomach to fuel the muscles of the endurance athlete during the later stages of the event. Drinks with higher concentrations of carbohydrates and electrolytes should be avoided, except near the end of exhaustive events, because they are retained in the stomach longer, not allowing the water and glucose to reach the tissues where they are needed.

Myth # 2: electrolyte solutions are needed to replace losses from perspiration.

Drinking electrolyte-laced beverages to replace fluid losses does not enhance athletic performance; minerals from the diet are sufficient to replenish stores after exercise. A pre-exercise carbohydrate beverage supplying glucose and/or fructose anytime preceding the sports activity helps to postpone exhaustion, and caffeine seems to give an extra boost to some in endurance events. Fruit juices can be used to supply the carbohydrates, provided they do not cause gastric distress. After exercise, the same carbohydrate/electrolyte beverage as mentioned earlier immediately following exercise gets the process of replenishing muscle glycogen and rehydrating the body underway quickly; glucose and sucrose are preferable to fructose. As above, a little sodium simply stimulates the absorption of the carbohydrate and water from the gut.

Homebrew Sports Drink: since many individuals are sensitive to the artificial colors and flavors often found in commercial sports drinks, try the following homemade sports drink: mix your favorite fruit juice with an equal portion of water and add one level teaspoon of salt for each quart. Drink well-chilled for faster absorption.

will allow you to be yourself. The release that you feel will smooth the rough spots in your life so that you can find more spontaneous delight in your sport.

Use breathing and asan techniques to contact your inner body. This will give you the power to make dependable, correct decisions.

Weight training strengthens your character by building a strong core of conditioning; you are strengthening muscles very deep inside the body. I think that the best thing that you could possibly do is to strengthen your body deep inside because that's where your core essence is. So not only are you getting your physical self in shape, but your spirituality, your mental strength is increased.

What we concentrate on is building the inner muscle groups so you are fit from the inside out. There's an essence of strength that exudes when you feel fit. People feel so much better about themselves when they have a strong feeling from the inside out.

—Tim Watnem

The Sport Routines

The exercises for strength sports focus on flexibility, a vital part of overall fitness for any athlete but especially for those whose sport demands extra strength training. For best results, always include a few minutes of breathing and meditation in your daily practice session.

Weight Training

Yoga exercises provide all-around flexibility training that will complement the deep muscle strengthening of weight training. Yoga breathing techniques help to oxygenate muscles fully and provide a solid foundation for rapid recovery from stress that otherwise lodges in muscle tissue as tension.

Muscles and joints can easily be stressed or injured by overexertion during weight training. The best way to prevent these injuries is working with a qualified trainer and using Yoga techniques for a thorough warm-up.

Modify your core routine as follows:

Complete Breath with Arm Circles

Add this exercise before the Shoulder Roll (pages 28–29). Sit in a comfortable position as described in Chapter 2, page 20. Begin the Complete Breath exercise, but add this component: as you breathe in, raise your arms in circles to the sides and over your head. At the top, hold your breath in for just a moment as you stretch up with your fists (Figure 8.1). Then breathe out as you lower your arms in a circle back to the floor. Repeat three to five times.

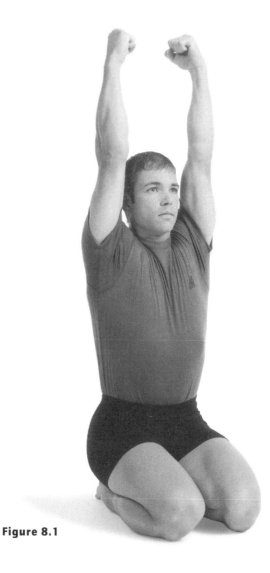

Figure 8.1

Lunge Series

Add this exercise between the Twisting Triangle and the Cat Breath (pages 33–34). With your toes pointed inward, spread your legs as far apart as you comfortably can. Breathe in as you turn completely toward the left and bend your left leg, bringing your left elbow underneath your left knee and resting on both fists (Figure 8.2). Keep your right leg straight if you can; if that position

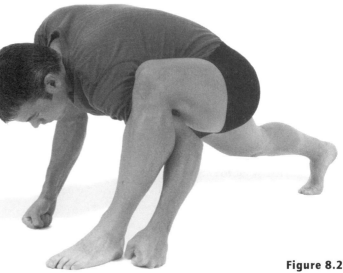

Figure 8.2

PROTEIN: TOO MUCH OF A GOOD THING

Food Myth # 1: athletes burn protein for extra energy.

The athlete's need for protein is not significantly greater than that for an inactive person, except during periods of increased-intensity endurance exercise and in the beginning stages of strength training. At these times, the protein requirement may double (or even triple in the latter case). Protein is used to repair and rebuild tissues throughout the body and to build up muscle tissue for greater strength, so for most sport-related activity, there is only a slight increase (50 percent above that of an inactive adult) needed to supply each day's new growth and repair. Normally the body does not use protein to provide fuel for exercise, with the exception of endurance events that are long enough to exhaust carbohydrate resources.

Only about 15 percent of daily calories should be in the form of protein, but most Americans already eat about twice as much protein as recommended and can benefit greatly from replacing some dietary protein with carbohydrate foods. This is also true for athletes. Protein consumed in excess of need must be excreted with water, which may contribute to dehydration.

Best Food Sources for Protein

The best foods provide protein without a lot of extra fat; greasy meats like steak, hamburgers, hot dogs, and fatty cheeses, etc., make poor choices. On the other hand, foods such as low-fat milk and yogurt, low-fat cheeses, tofu, lentils, peas, and beans are all excellent choices. Nutritional yeast is 23 percent protein, so even a 1-oz serving provides as much as a cup of milk. Non-vegetarians can replace these high-protein foods with 4 to 6 oz of meat, fish, or poultry. Care should be taken to eliminate the usual accompanying fat.

The Great Protein Myth

Food Myth # 2: extra protein builds bigger, stronger muscles. Eating protein does not build muscle; exercise does! The muscle-building process is fueled by carbohydrates, which are used to work the muscles, with only small amounts of protein required to build strength by adding muscle tissue. The hardest-training body builder needs only 50 percent more protein, except when first beginning weight training. Endurance athletes may need double protein for a month or so when beginning or significantly increasing their exercise load.

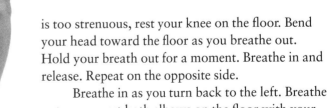

Figure 8.3

is too strenuous, rest your knee on the floor. Bend your head toward the floor as you breathe out. Hold your breath out for a moment. Breathe in and release. Repeat on the opposite side.

Breathe in as you turn back to the left. Breathe out as you rest both elbows on the floor with your left elbow inside your left knee, lower your right knee to the floor, clasp your hands, and bend your head toward your hands (Figure 8.3). Hold your breath out for a moment.

Breathe in as you push yourself up, rest your left arm on your left thigh, and straighten your right arm and your right leg (Figure 8.4). Breathe out and hold your breath out for a moment.

Breathe in and release. With your legs in the same position, breathe out as you stretch both arms out to the sides, resting your chest on your left thigh (Figure 8.5). Hold your breath out for a moment.

Bring your left hand to the floor on the inside of your left leg. Breathe in and stretch your right arm straight up toward the ceiling (Figure 8.6). Look at your outstretched fingers and hold your breath in for a moment.

Breathe out, bring your arm down, swivel over to the right, and repeat the series facing right.

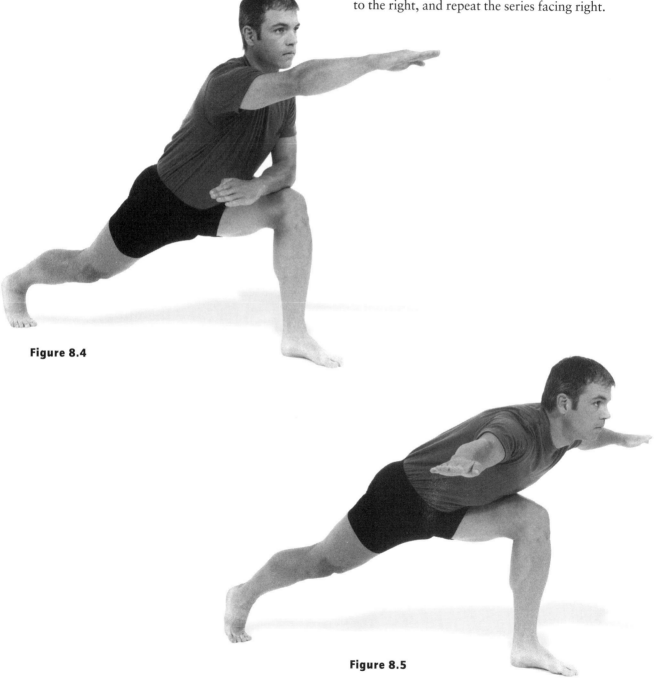

Figure 8.4

Figure 8.5

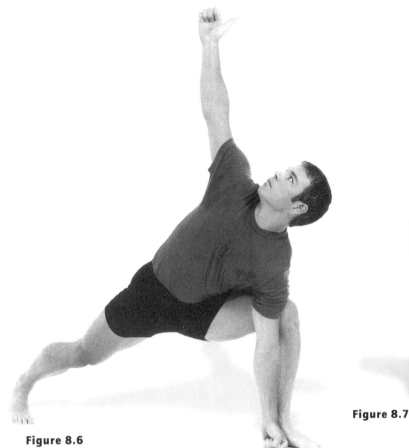

Figure 8.6

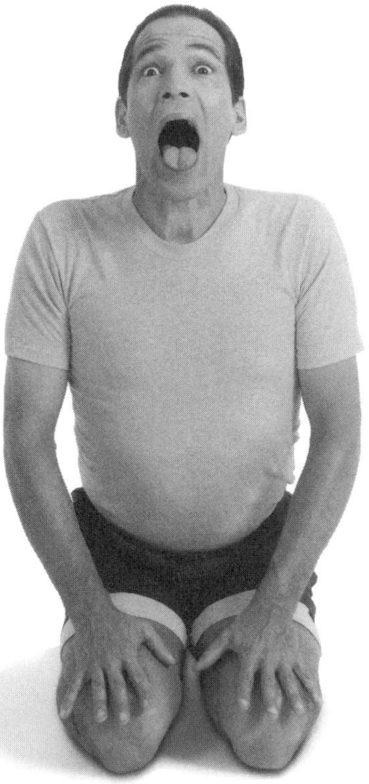

Figure 8.7

Camel Pose (pictured, page 151)

Add this exercise between the Cat Breath and the Cobra V-Raise (page 34). From a kneeling position, separate your knees slightly, arch your back, and grasp your left heel with your left hand. Breathe normally. Do this once on each side to warm up. Then reach back and grasp both heels. Push your hips forward as far as possible without straining. Let your head gently fall back as you breathe out (unless you have a disk problem in your upper back or neck, in which case keep your head up).

    Variation: if you are unable to grasp both heels at once, do the exercise once on each side in the beginning position instead.

Lion Pose

Add the next three exercises between the Baby Pose and the Cobra Pose (pages 34–35). Sit on your feet, or cross-legged. Spread your fingers apart like a

lion's paws and grip your knees. Lean forward slightly and take a deep breath through your nose. Open your eyes wide, raise your eyebrows, stick out your tongue, and roar fiercely like a lion (Figure 8.7). Visualize and try to look like a roaring lion.

Pigeon Pose

From a kneeling position, slide your right leg back so you are sitting on your left foot. Your right leg should be as straight as possible, knee to the floor. Place your hands on either side of your left knee and your forehead on the floor (Figure 8.8). Breathe out

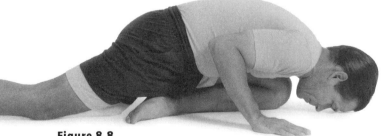

Figure 8.8

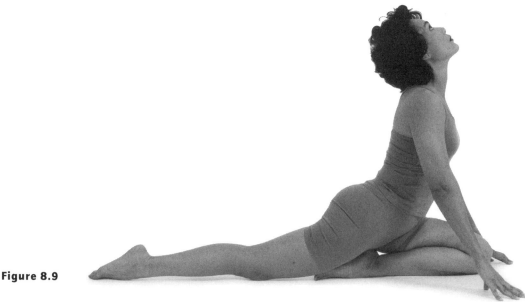

Figure 8.9

completely, then breathe in as you curl up, head first, then chest, then stomach, curling back as far as you can. You can press up on your fingertips for an extra stretch (Figure 8.9). Look up toward your forehead. Hold your breath in for a moment. Breathe out and curl down, stomach first, keeping your head and eyes up until your head reaches the floor. Repeat three times.

Then push yourself up on your fists, straighten your arms, relax your back, and stare at one spot on the floor about three feet in front of you (Figure 8.10). Breathe out and hold. Breathe in as you release the position.

Alternate Seated Sun Pose

Sit with legs outstretched. Bend your left knee and place your foot on the inside of your right thigh (Figure 8.11). Breathe in and bring your arms in a wide circle to the sides and over your head (Figure 8.12). Stretch from the rib cage and look up. Hold your breath in for a moment. Breathe out and bend forward over your outstretched leg, keeping your toes flexed. Grasp your ankle or foot with both hands, bend your elbows, and pull your torso gently toward your left leg (Figure 8.13). Hold your breath out for a moment. (*Note:* if you are limber enough to reach

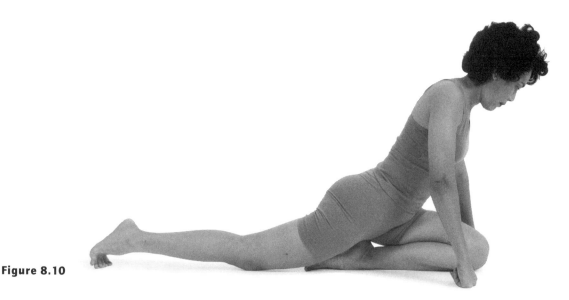

Figure 8.10

your foot and still bend your elbows, grasp the big toe with both hands, as shown in Figure 8.14.)

Breathe in and raise your arms to the sides and over your head again. Stretch and look up. Hold your breath in for a moment. Breathe out and lower. Repeat three times. Repeat on the opposite side.

Note: if you are limber enough so that your bent knee touches the floor when you place your foot on top of the opposite thigh instead of inside, you may do the exercise in this position. To increase limberness in your knee and hip, place your foot on top of the opposite thigh and gently press down on the upraised knee with your hand, as in Figure 8.15. Support yourself by leaning on your opposite hand.

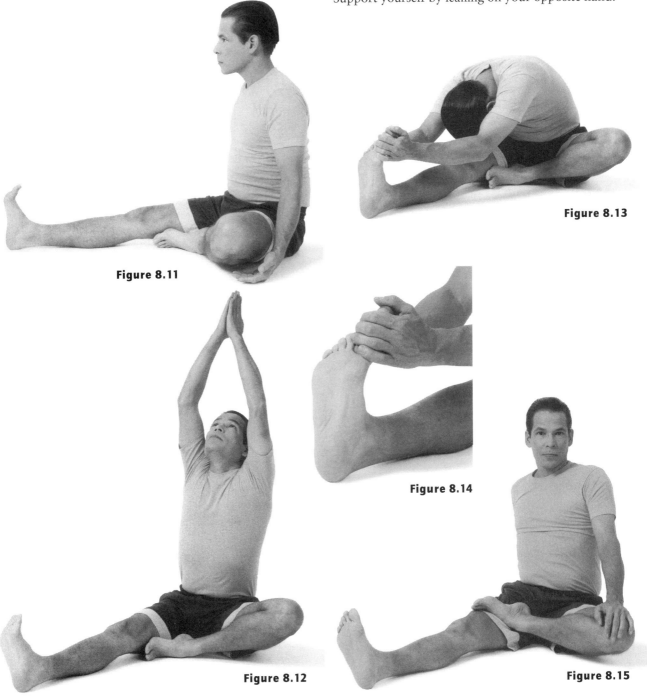

Figure 8.11

Figure 8.13

Figure 8.12

Figure 8.14

Figure 8.15

Boat Pose (pictured, page 161)

Add this exercise between the Cobra Pose and the Knee Squeeze (pages 35–36). Lying on your stomach, stretch your arms on the floor over your head and place your forehead on the floor. Breathe out. Breathe in as you lift your arms, legs, and head, looking up through your forehead. Hold your breath in for a moment. Breathe out and release, bringing your arms and forehead back to the floor. Repeat twice more.

Plow Pose (pictured, page 152–153)

Add this exercise after the Knee Squeeze (page 36). From a seated position, bend your knees and roll back and forth once or twice. Then roll back onto your shoulders, bringing your knees to your forehead and supporting your back with your hands. Breathe in, hold a moment, then breathe out, extending your legs behind your head, carefully trying to touch your toes to the floor. Breathe naturally and hold the position for several seconds.

If you wish, try this variation: straighten your arms on the floor over your head and hold for several seconds.

Breathe in and bend your knees back to your forehead, supporting your back with your hands, then roll forward to a cross-legged position, stretching your head and arms forward. Breathe naturally as you rest for about 10 seconds.

Note: if you have a disk problem in your neck or upper back, do not do this exercise; substitute the Easy Bridge (page 78).

Wrestling

To prepare fully for the short intense burst of activity in wrestling, use Yoga exercises to thoroughly warm up all the muscle groups and build flexibility, especially in the shoulders and upper back. Breathing techniques will help build stamina, and meditation and fantasy techniques can be used to build focus and strength. Wrestlers are prone to eating disorders; see "Abnormal Eating Patterns" on page 127.

Most injuries in wrestling occur due to levered force rather than sudden impact. The most common areas for muscle strains are the neck, shoulder, and elbow.

> *You have to think in a wrestling match, but I guess some of this fits into the whole idea of thinking with another part of your brain, and perhaps even a mystical kind of thought. You almost have to allow your mind to talk to your body. Obviously you can't sit there and literally think through every move. But somehow your mind does do it and your body reacts. When I'm wrestling it's almost like a trance state where some other part of who I am is in control of what I am doing because of the complexity of what's happening physically and mentally. Something else seems to be doing the wrestling. Emotionally that makes me feel very centered, very in tune with another part of myself.*
>
> —Nelson Gonzalez

Modify your core routine as follows:

Complete Breath with Arm Circles (pictured, page 138)

Add this exercise before the Shoulder Roll (pages 28–29). Sit in a comfortable position as described in Chapter 2, page 20. Begin the Complete Breath exercise, but add this component: as you breathe in, raise your arms in circles to the sides and over your head. At the top, hold your breath in for just a moment as you stretch up with your fists. Then breathe out as you lower your arms in a circle back to the floor. Repeat three to five times.

Dancer Pose and Extension

Add this exercise between the Standing Sun Pose and the Hip Rotation (pages 31–32). From a standing position, bend your left leg back and grasp your left foot with your right hand (Figure 8.16). Throughout the exercise, steady yourself by fixing your gaze on one spot on the wall in front of you. Slowly move into the completed Dancer Pose by raising your left arm straight up toward the ceiling and pulling your lifted leg up and back as far as possible without strain (Figure 8.17). Keep your right (supporting) leg straight and keep your gaze focused on one spot. Breathe in and hold your breath in for a moment.

Figure 8.16

Maintaining your gaze, slowly breathe out and lower your body into the extended position (Figure 8.18). Keep your lifted leg as far up and back as possible. Your left arm extends straight ahead. Your supporting leg remains straight. Stare at one spot for balance. Don't strain. Hold for a moment, then breathe in, come back to a standing position, and switch sides.

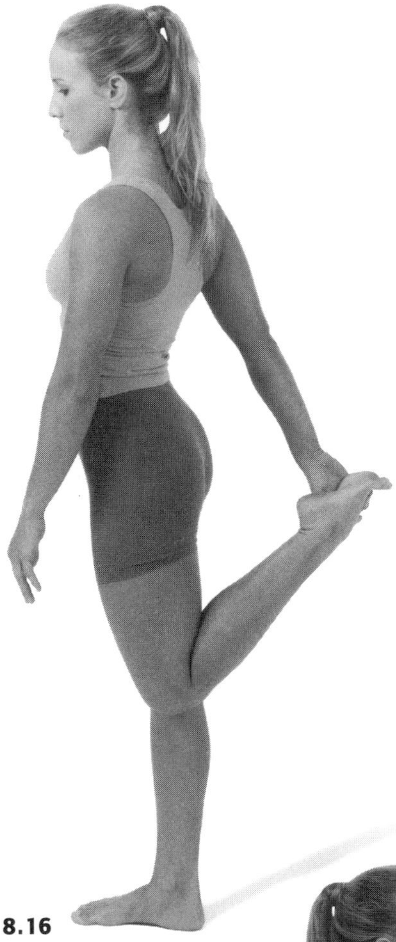

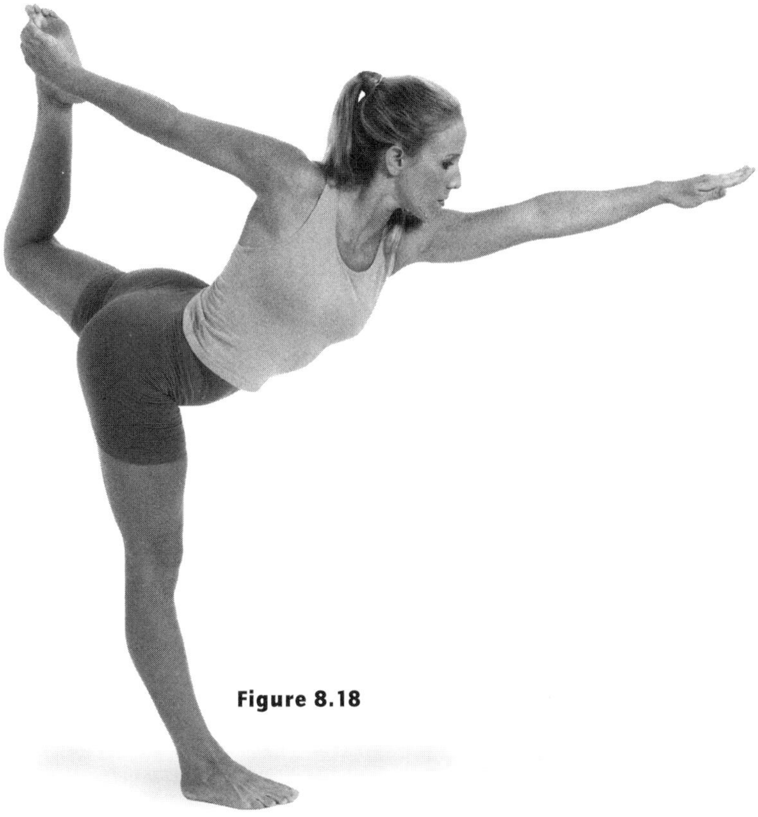

Figure 8.18

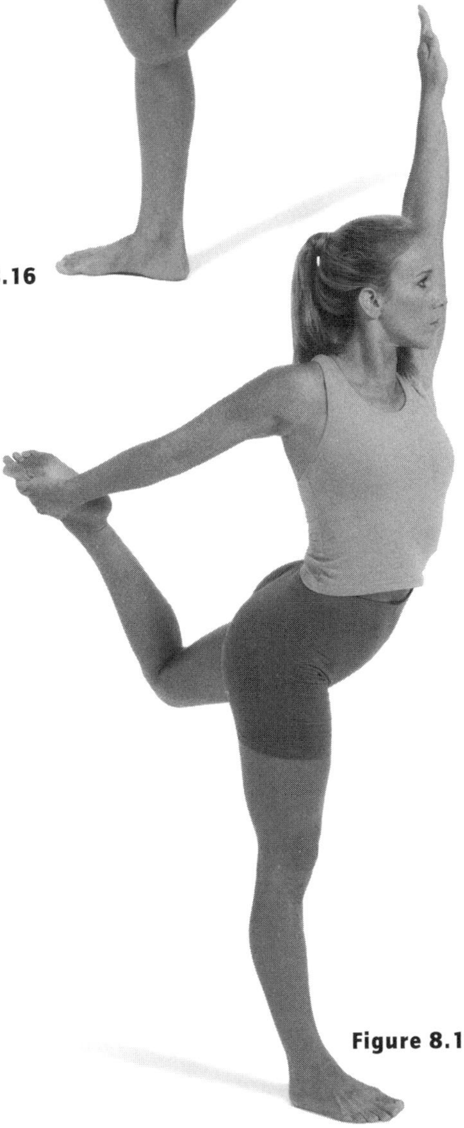

Figure 8.17

T Pose (pictured, page 154)

Add the next two exercises between the Twisting Triangle and the Cat Breath (pages 33–34). When you are first learning this position, stand three to four feet from a chair or other support. Lean forward and hold on to the support with both hands. Lift your left leg in back as high as you can, ideally, parallel to the floor. Alternatively, brace yourself with both hands on the knee of your supporting leg. Keep your right (supporting) leg straight. Your torso and left leg should be in a straight line parallel to the floor. Keep your neck straight, breathe naturally, and look at a spot on the floor.

When you feel steady, release your grip on the support and place your palms together, pushing your arms out parallel to the floor. Relax your breath. Look forward at your hands. Lower your leg and return to a standing position. Rest until your breath returns to normal. Repeat on the opposite side.

Warrior Pose (pictured, page 155)

When you are strong enough, you can perform this exercise immediately after the T Pose on one side, then repeat both exercises on the opposite side.

Place both hands on your right knee and lift your left leg straight in back. Bend your right knee and let your torso rest on your right thigh as you slide your hands down to support either side of your right ankle. Keep your left leg high in back. Tuck your head. Breathe out and hold your breath out for a moment. Breathe in, slowly release, and repeat on opposite side.

Variation: lace your fingers behind your back. If you can, lock your elbows, squeezing your shoulder blades together. Lift one leg as high as possible, bend your supporting leg, rest your chest on your thigh if possible, and lift your arms away from your back. Breathe out and hold for a moment. Release and switch sides.

Bow Variation

Add the next three exercises between the Cat Breath and the Cobra V-Raise (page 34). Start on your

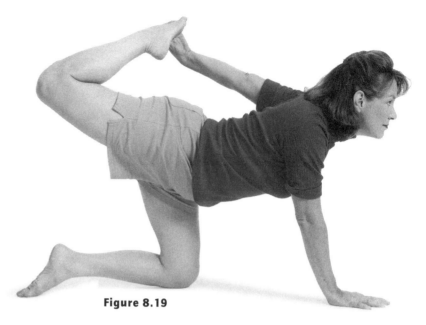

Figure 8.19

hands and knees. Reach back with your left hand and grasp your right foot. Stare at one spot on the wall or floor for balance as you breathe in and lift your foot up and away from your body as far as possible (Figure 8.19). Hold your breath in for a moment. Breathe out, release slowly, and switch sides. Repeat three times on each side.

Lion Pose (pictured, page 141)

Sit on your feet, or cross-legged. Spread your fingers apart like a lion's paws and grip your knees. Lean forward slightly and take a deep breath through your nose. Open your eyes wide, raise your eyebrows, stick out your tongue, and roar fiercely like a lion. Visualize and try to look like a roaring lion.

Pigeon Pose (pictured, pages 141–142)

From a kneeling position, slide your right leg back so you are sitting on your left foot. Your right leg should be as straight as possible, knee to the floor. Place your hands on either side of your left knee and your forehead on the floor. Breathe out completely, then breathe in as you curl up, head first, then chest, then stomach, curling back as far as you can. You can press up on your fingertips for an extra stretch. Look up toward your forehead. Hold your breath in for a moment. Breathe out and curl down, stomach first, keeping your head and eyes up until your head reaches the floor. Repeat three times.

Then push yourself up on your fists, straighten your arms, relax your back, and stare at one spot on the floor about three feet in front of you. Breathe out and hold. Breathe in as you release the position.

Seated Sun Pose and Alternate
(pictured, pages 86–87)

Add this exercise between the Baby Pose and the Cobra Pose (pages 34–35). Bring both legs straight out in front of you and flex your toes. Sit straight, breathe out with your arms at your sides, then breathe in as you raise your arms in a wide circle to the sides and overhead. Press your palms together, look up, visualize the sun, and stretch from the rib cage. Hold your breath in for a moment.

Breathe out as you bend forward, tucking your chin toward your chest. Grasp your ankles, bend your elbows, and pull your torso toward your legs (remember to pull by bending your arms, not by pushing with your lower back). Hold your breath out for a moment.

If you are limber enough to reach your feet (and still bend your elbows), grasp your big toes as shown on page 86.

Release and breathe in, bringing your arms to the sides and over your head again. Stretch and look up as before. Breathe out and bring your arms back down to your sides. Repeat three times.

Alternate Seated Sun Pose: sit with legs outstretched. Bend your left knee and place your foot on the inside of your right thigh. Breathe in and bring your arms in a wide circle to the sides and over your

head. Stretch from the rib cage and look up. Hold your breath in for a moment. Breathe out and bend forward over your outstretched leg, keeping your toes flexed. Grasp your ankle or foot with both hands, bend your elbows, and pull your torso gently toward your left leg. Hold your breath out for a moment. (*Note:* if you are limber enough to reach your foot and still bend your elbows, grasp the big toe with both hands, as shown on page 87.)

Breathe in and raise your arms to the sides and over your head again. Stretch and look up. Hold your breath in for a moment. Breathe out and lower. Repeat three times. Repeat on the opposite side.

Note: if you are limber enough so that your bent knee touches the floor when you place your foot on top of the opposite thigh instead of inside, you may do the exercise in this position. To increase limberness in your knee and hip, place your foot on top of the opposite thigh and gently press down on the upraised knee with your hand. Support yourself by leaning on your opposite hand, as shown on page 87.

Bow Pose

Add this exercise between the Cobra Pose and the Knee Squeeze (pages 35–36). Lie on your stomach with your forehead to the floor. Bend your knees and grasp your ankles or feet with your hands (Figure 8.20; you may have to separate your legs slightly to reach). Breathe in as you lift and look up, pulling up on your feet so you balance on your stomach (Figure 8.21). Look up through your forehead. Hold

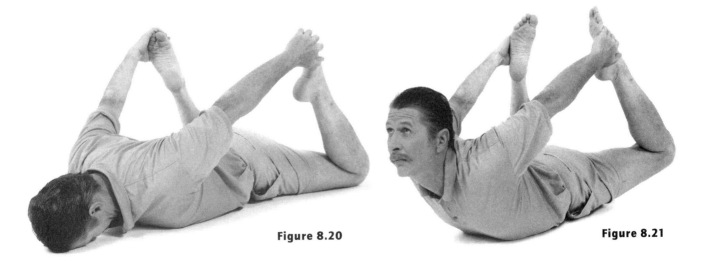

Figure 8.20   **Figure 8.21**

your breath in for a moment. Breathe out and release. Repeat twice more.

Shoulder Stand

Add this exercise after the Knee Squeeze (page 36). Do not do this exercise if you have back or neck problems; substitute the Easy Bridge (page 163).

In a seated position with your knees bent and your arms around your knees (Figure 8.22), roll back and forth a few times (Figure 8.23), then roll back onto your shoulders, immediately supporting your back with your hands (Figure 8.24) and keeping your knees bent and touching your forehead (Figure 8.25).

Slowly straighten your legs toward the ceiling and push your back straighter by using your hands (Figure 8.26). Stare at the spot between your big toes and breathe out. Hold your breath out for a moment. Breathe in and relax your breath.

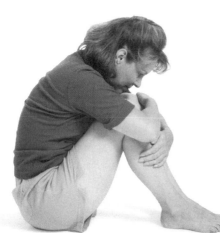

Figure 8.22

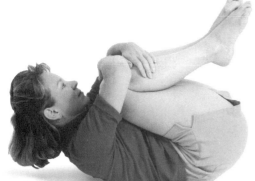

Figure 8.23

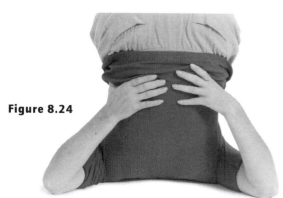

Figure 8.24

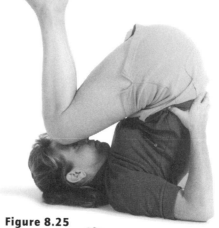

Figure 8.25

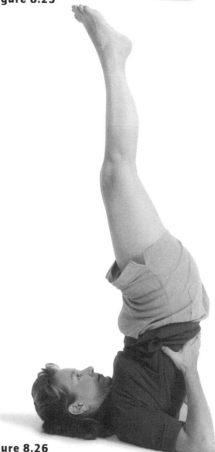

Figure 8.26

MAGIC POTIONS: MOSTLY WORTHLESS, GENERALLY NOT HARMFUL

Products claiming to be magic bullets deluge athletes and coaches. Marketers unrelentingly exploit your search for a competitive edge. In a never-ending quest, athletes have tried quick fixes, from the mundane to the bizarre. Here is a partial list of those now found to be ineffective:

Bee pollen
Seaweed
Freeze-dried liver flakes
Gelatin
Amino acid supplements
Ginseng
Dimethylglycine (DMG)
Pangamate
Inosine (actually detrimental!)

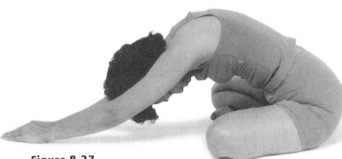

Figure 8.27

Bend your knees back to your forehead, supporting your back with your hands, then roll forward into a cross-legged position, reaching your head and arms forward (Figure 8.27). Breathe naturally as you rest for at least 10 seconds.

Martial Arts

Originating as a means of self-defense, the martial arts have evolved into sports in which the mental aspect is as important as the physical. Yoga can help in all three areas of practice: yoga exercises that emphasize balance, coordination, and strength will build concentration, muscle tone, and erect posture. Breathing techniques will improve stamina, focus, and reaction time. Meditation training will open you to the intuitive voice of the inner self to better anticipate your opponent's movements.

Common injuries among martial artists include "runner's knee" due to bent knee position, contact injuries, and knee and other joint injuries from rapid shifts in position. The best way to prevent these injuries is through all-around flexibility training and strengthening the legs and joints.

Modify your core routine as follows:

Dancer Pose and Extension
(pictured, page 145)
Add the next two exercises between the Standing Sun Pose and the Hip Rotation (pages 31–32). From a standing position, bend your left leg back and grasp your left foot with your right hand. Throughout the exercise, steady yourself by fixing your gaze on one spot on the wall in front of you. Slowly move into the completed Dancer Pose by raising your left arm straight up toward the ceiling and pulling your lifted leg up and back as far as possible without strain. Keep your right (supporting) leg straight and keep your gaze focused on one spot. Breathe in and hold your breath in for a moment.

Maintaining your gaze, slowly breathe out and lower your body into the extended position. Keep your lifted leg as far up and back as possible. Your left arm extends straight ahead. Your supporting leg remains straight. Stare at one spot for balance. Don't strain. Hold for a moment, then breathe in, come back to a standing position, and switch sides.

Tree Pose
From a standing position, lift your right foot and place it on the inside of your left thigh (Figure 8.28). Relax the leg to help hold your foot in position. Bare feet will also help. If you feel unsteady, hold on to a sturdy chair. Steady yourself by gazing at one spot on the wall or floor without bending your neck. Breathe in as you raise your arms slowly over your head, straighten your arms, and place your palms together (Figure 8.29). Hold your breath in for a moment. Breathe out and bring your arms and leg down slowly. Repeat on the opposite side.

be in a straight line parallel to the floor. Keep your neck straight, breathe naturally, and look at a spot on the floor.

When you feel steady, release your grip on the support and place your palms together, pushing your arms out parallel to the floor. Relax your breath. Look forward at your hands. Lower your leg and return to a standing position. Rest until your breath returns to normal. Repeat on the opposite side.

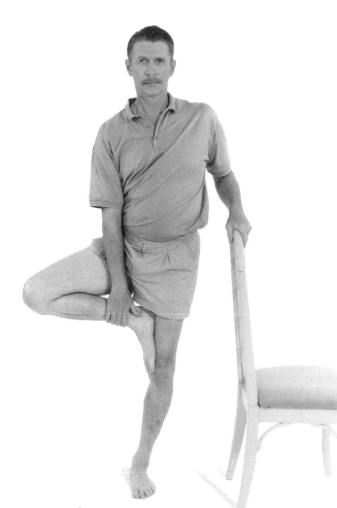

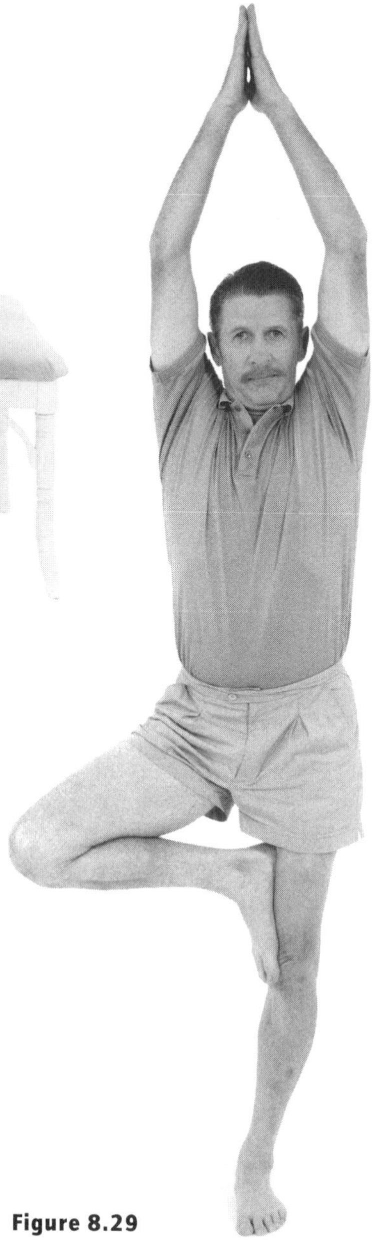

Figure 8.28

If you are limber enough, you may place your foot on top of your thigh for this exercise (Figure 8.30).

T Pose (pictured, page 154)
Add this exercise between the Twisting Triangle and the Cat Breath (pages 33–34). When you are first learning this exercise, stand three to four feet from a chair or other support. Lean forward and hold on to the support with both hands. Lift your left leg in back as high as you can, ideally, parallel to the floor. Alternatively, brace yourself with both hands on the knee of your supporting leg. Keep your right (supporting) leg straight. Your torso and left leg should

Figure 8.29 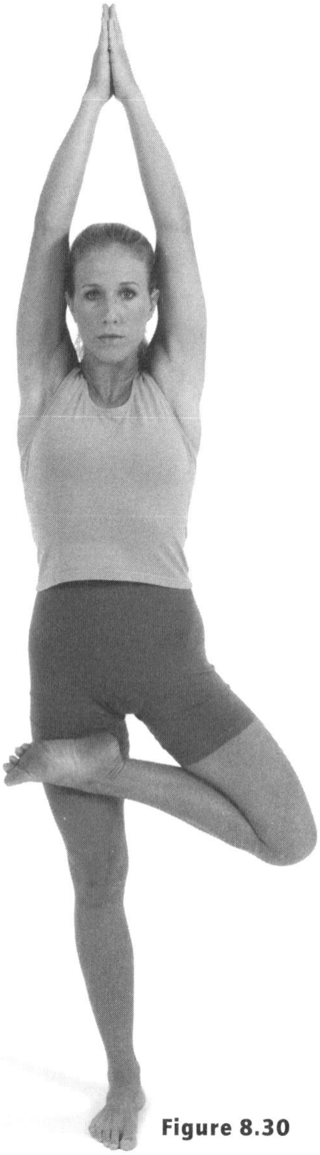 **Figure 8.30**

Bow Variation (pictured, page 146)

Add the next two exercises between the Cat Breath and the Cobra V-Raise (page 34). Start on your hands and knees. Reach back with your left hand and grasp your right foot. Stare at one spot on the wall or floor for balance as you breathe in and lift your foot up and away from your body as far as possible. Hold your breath in for a moment. Breathe out, release slowly, and switch sides. Repeat three times on each side.

Camel Pose

From a kneeling position, separate your knees slightly, arch your back, and grasp your left heel with your left hand (Figure 8.31). Breathe normally. Do this once on each side to warm up. Then reach back and grasp both heels (Figure 8.32). Push your hips forward as far as possible without straining. Let your head gently fall back as you breathe out (unless you have a disk problem in your upper back or neck, in which case keep your head up).

Variation: if you are unable to grasp both heels at once, do the exercise once on each side in the beginning position instead.

Lion Pose (pictured, page 141)

Add this exercise between the Baby Pose and the Cobra Pose (pages 34–35). Sit on your feet, or cross-legged. Spread your fingers apart like a lion's paws and grip your knees. Lean forward slightly and take a deep breath through your nose. Open your eyes wide, raise your eyebrows, stick out your tongue, and roar fiercely like a lion. Visualize and try to look like a roaring lion.

Shoulder Stand and Plow (Shoulder Stand pictured, page 148)

Add these exercises after the Knee Squeeze (page 36). Do not do this exercise if you have back or neck problems; substitute the Easy Bridge (page 163).

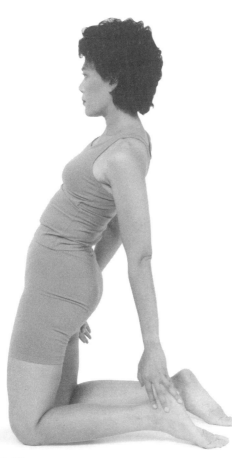

Figure 8.31

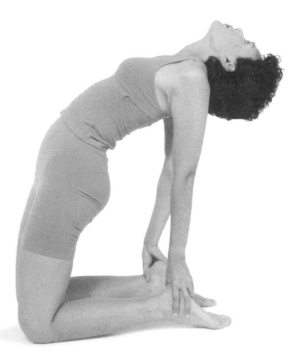

Figure 8.32

In a seated position with knees bent and arms around your knees, roll back and forth a few times, then roll back onto your shoulders; immediately supporting your back with your hands and keeping your knees bent and touching your forehead.

Slowly straighten your legs toward the ceiling and push your back straighter by using your hands. Stare at the spot between your big toes and breathe out. Hold your breath out for a moment. Breathe in and relax your breath.

Bring your knees back to your forehead, supporting your back with your hands. Breathe in, hold a moment, then breathe out, extending your legs behind your head, carefully trying to touch your toes to the floor (Figure 8.33). Breathe naturally and hold the position for several seconds.

If you wish, try this variation: straighten your arms on the floor over your head and hold for several seconds (Figure 8.34).

Making Weight

Wrestlers and body builders often restrict food and fluid intake to certify for a weight classification that is well below their off-season weight, and are prone to rapid and large cycles of weight loss and regain. Methods commonly used to lose weight are dehydration through the use of saunas, rubber suits, fluid restriction, severe low-calorie diets, fasting, and purging by vomiting and the use of laxatives and diuretics. These practices produce fatigue and have a negative effect on performance as well as normal growth. (See sidebar on abnormal eating patterns, page 127, for additional cautions.)

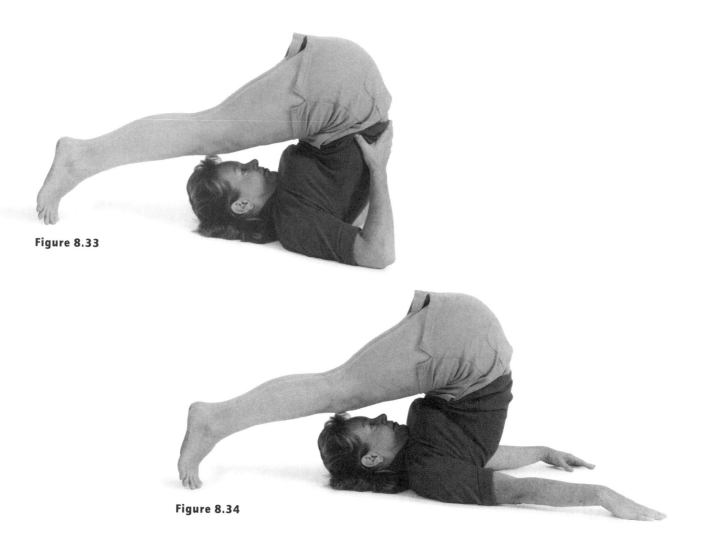

Figure 8.33

Figure 8.34

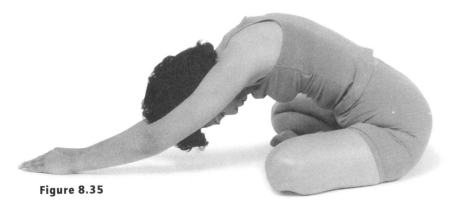

Figure 8.35

Breathe in and bend your knees back to your forehead, supporting your back with your hands, then roll forward to a cross-legged position, stretching your head and arms forward (Figure 8.35). Breathe naturally as you rest for at least 10 seconds.

Surfing/Sailboarding

Surfing demands unusual skills of balance, timing, and coordination. Board-sailing (or wind-surfing) gives the athlete slightly more control than a surfer has. Both sports can be enhanced with the balance, flexibility, and strengthening qualities of many Yoga exercises. Breathing and meditation will improve focus and stamina. You can also use fantasy to improve your technique when you're not on the water.

Shoulder and elbow stress from constant pull on the sail is a common problem in board-sailing; falls are a problem for fans of both sports. The best way to prevent these injuries is to strengthen the upper and lower body, to improve balance and concentration, and through overall conditioning.

Modify your core routine as follows:

Tree Pose (pictured, page 150)

Add the next two exercises between the Standing Sun Pose and the Hip Rotation (pages 31–32). From a standing position, lift your right foot and place it on the inside of your left thigh. Relax the leg to help hold your foot in position. Bare feet will also help. If you feel unsteady, hold on to a sturdy chair. Steady yourself by gazing at one spot on the wall or floor without bending your neck. Breathe in as you raise your arms slowly over your head, straighten your arms, and place your palms together. Hold your breath in for a moment. Breathe out and bring your arms and leg down slowly. Repeat on the opposite side.

If you are limber enough, you may place your foot on top of your thigh for this exercise.

Archer Pose (pictured, pages 158–159)

Place your right foot directly in front of the left, both pointed straight ahead. If you feel unsteady in this position, you may separate your feet slightly at first, but both should point forward. Extend your left arm straight ahead and position the hand as if you were holding a bow, with the thumb pointed up. Place your right hand on your head with fingers curled to hold the string of the bow.

Breathe in, looking forward at your thumb, then slowly and carefully breathe out and turn toward the left, keeping your left arm outstretched and following your thumb with your gaze. Twist back as far as you can and stare at your thumb. Hold your breath out for a moment.

Breathe in as you twist slowly back to face front. Relax your arms and your breath. Keeping your feet in the same position, switch the positions of your arms (right hand outstretched, left hand on your head). Stare at the thumb of your outstretched hand. Breathe in, then slowly and carefully twist back to the right this time, breathing out. Hold your breath out for a moment, staring at your thumb.

Repeat the sequence with your left foot forward.

T Pose

Add the next two exercises between the Twisting Triangle and the Cat Breath (pages 33–34). When you are first learning this exercise, stand three to four feet from a chair or other support. Lean forward and hold on to the support with both hands. Lift your left leg in back as high as you can (Figure 8.36), ideally, parallel to the floor. Alternatively, brace yourself with both hands on the knee of your supporting leg (Figure 8.37). Keep your right (supporting) leg straight. Your torso and left leg should be in a straight line parallel to the floor. Keep your neck straight, breathe naturally, and look at a spot on the floor.

When you feel steady, release your grip on the support and place your palms together, pushing your

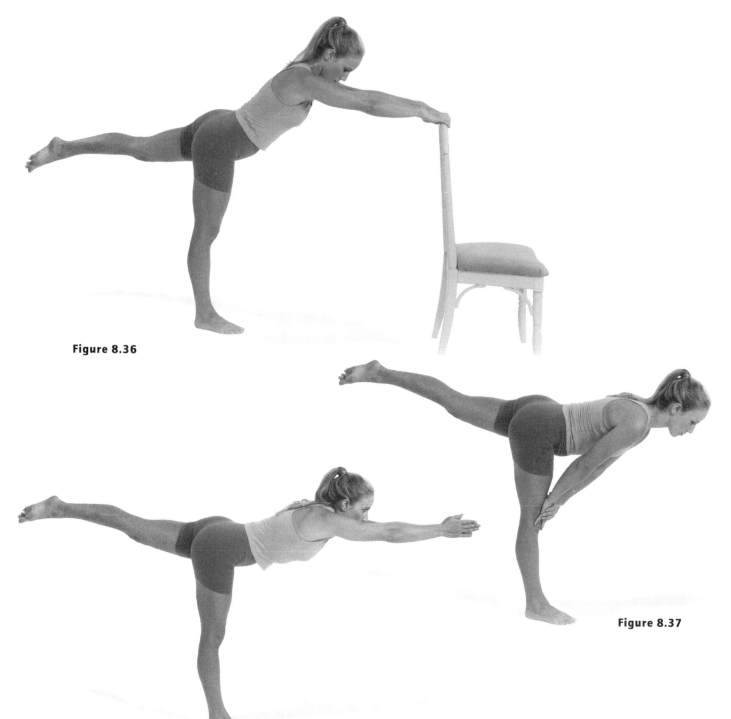

Figure 8.36

Figure 8.37

Figure 8.38

arms out parallel to the floor (Figure 8.38). Relax your breath. Look forward at your hands. Lower your leg and return to a standing position. Rest until your breath returns to normal. Repeat on the opposite side.

Warrior Pose

When you are strong enough, you can perform this exercise immediately after the T Pose on one side, then repeat both exercises on the opposite side.

Place both hands on your right knee and lift your left leg straight in back. Bend your right knee and let your torso rest on your right thigh as you

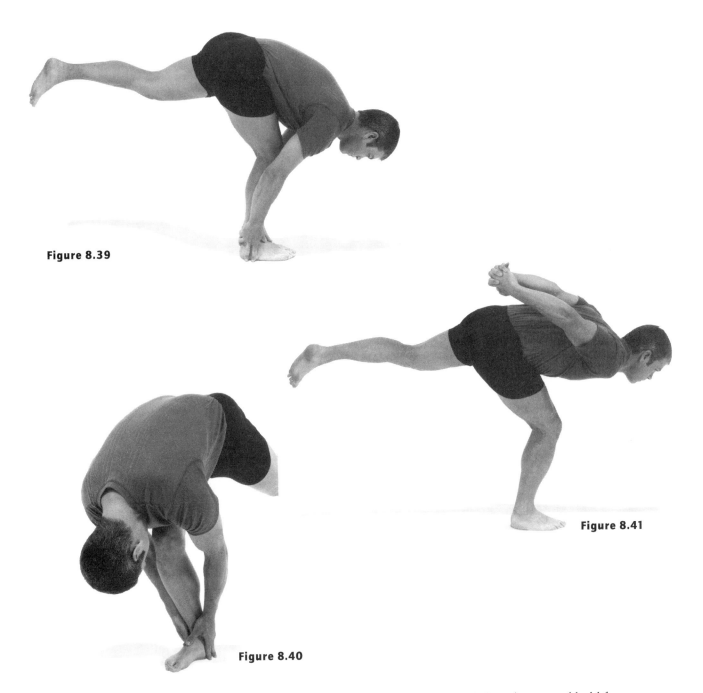

Figure 8.39

Figure 8.40

Figure 8.41

slide your hands down to support either side of your right ankle (Figures 8.39 and 8.40). Keep your left leg high in back. Tuck your head. Breathe out and hold your breath out for a moment. Breathe in, slowly release, and repeat on the opposite side.

Variation: lace your fingers behind your back. If you can, lock your elbows, squeezing your shoulder blades together. Lift one leg as high as possible, bend your supporting leg, rest your chest on your thigh if possible, and lift your arms away from your

back (Figure 8.41). Breathe out and hold for a moment. Release and switch sides.

Arm and Leg Balance

Add this exercise between the Cat Breath and the Cobra V-Raise (page 34). Start on your hands and knees. Breathe out completely, then breathe in as you lift your left arm and right leg (opposites) parallel to the floor (Figure 8.42). Stare at one spot and hold your breath in for a moment. Breathe out, release,

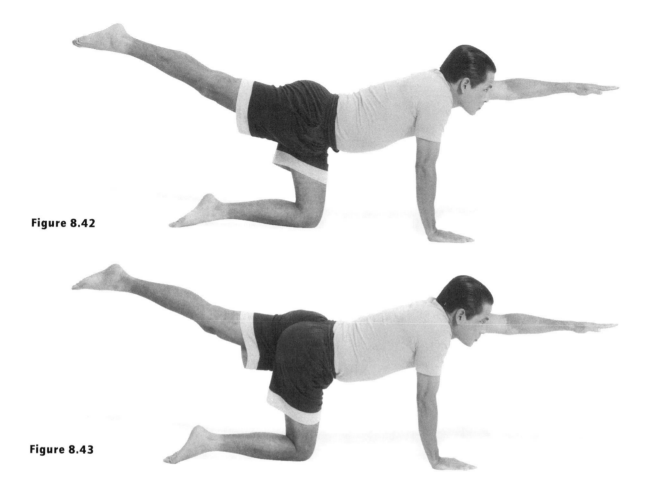

Figure 8.42

Figure 8.43

and repeat with the opposite arm and leg. Repeat three times on each side.

    Variation: lift the arm and leg on the same side of the body (Figure 8.43).

Plank Pose

Add this exercise between the Cobra V-Raise *and the* Baby Pose *(pages 34–35).* From a hands-and-knees position, straighten your legs out behind you, supporting yourself on your hands. Raise your hips and lower your shoulders until your body is in a straight line supported on your hands and feet (Figure 8.44). Shift your weight to your right arm and breathe in as you lift your left arm straight in front of you (Figure 8.45). Focus your gaze on your outstretched hand. Hold your breath in for a moment. Breathe out and release.

    Still supporting yourself on your right arm, breathe in as you bring your left arm to the side and up toward the ceiling (Figure 8.46). This will twist

ANTIOXIDANTS FOR RECOVERY AND LONG-TERM PROTECTION

It is well known that intense activity, urban ozone exposure, and high-altitude exercise all contribute to tissue damage due to free radicals. Antioxidant vitamins and minerals are the athlete's best bet to enhance long-term health by protecting against the adverse effects of these chemicals. Try the following daily antioxidant plan:

Vitamin E (d-a-tocopherol)	400–800 IU
Beta-carotene	25,000–100,000 IU
Vitamin C (ascorbate)	0.5–2 gr
Selenium (sodium selenite)	100–250 mcg

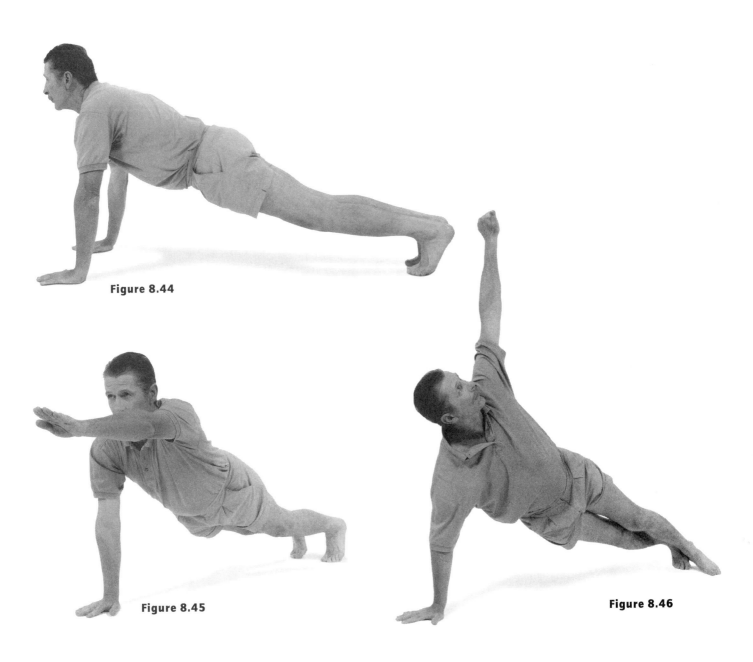

Figure 8.44

Figure 8.45

Figure 8.46

your body to the left as well. Look up toward your hand. Hold your breath in for a moment. Breathe out, bring your left hand down to the floor, and repeat the sequence on the opposite side. Then rest lying on your stomach.

Side Stretch (pictured, page 163)

Add this exercise between the Baby Pose and the Cobra Pose (pages 34–35). Sit up in a comfortable cross-legged position. Breathe in, then breathe out as you lean to the right and stretch your left arm up over your head and toward the right, stretching the entire left side of your torso. Hold your breath out

for a moment. Breathe in as you release, then repeat on the opposite side.

Skiing (Downhill)

Skiing demands quick reflexes, strong legs and back, and a healthy cardiovascular system; the sport is not unlike a sprint. A varied Yoga routine can provide flexibility and strength training, as well as a strong heart and lungs. Breathing and meditation techniques will improve concentration and stamina, and visualization exercises can be used to practice one's form mentally.

Downhill skiers often experience "runner's knee" from twists and turns in bent-knee position, and falls. Cross-training with in-line skating can help strengthen legs and joints in the off-season. General flexibility and strength training can help prepare skiers for the twists and turns of a downhill course and help prevent injury. Emphasize knee and leg-strengthening exercises to support the bent-knee position and reduce strain on the lower back.

Modify your core routine as follows:

Archer Pose

Add this exercise between the Standing Sun Pose and the Hip Rotation (pages 31–32). Place your right foot directly in front of the left, both pointed straight ahead. If you feel unsteady in this position, you may separate your feet slightly at first, but both should point forward. Extend your left arm straight ahead and position the hand as if you were holding a bow, with the thumb pointed up. Place your right hand on your head with fingers curled to hold the string of the bow (Figure 8.47).

Breathe in, looking forward at your thumb, then slowly and carefully breathe out and turn toward the left, keeping your left arm outstretched and following your thumb with your gaze. Twist back as far as you can and stare at your thumb (Figure 8.48). Hold your breath out for a moment.

Breathe in as you twist slowly back to face front. Relax your arms and your breath. Keeping your feet in the same position, switch the positions of your arms (right hand outstretched, left hand on your head). Stare at the thumb of your outstretched hand. Breathe in, then slowly and carefully twist

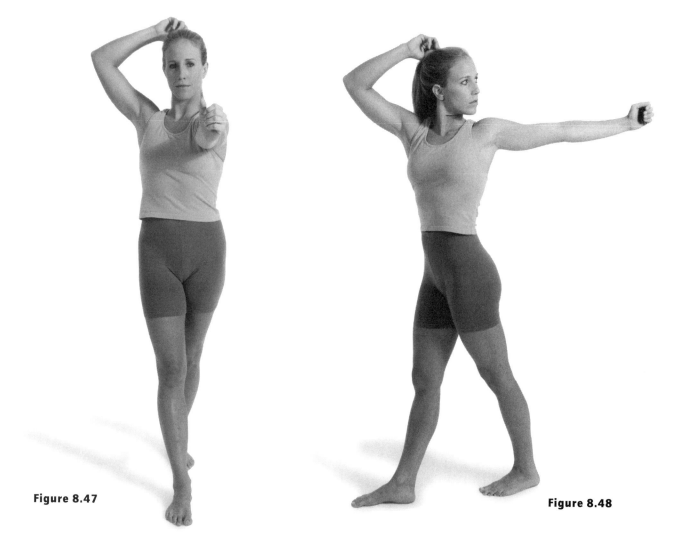

Figure 8.47   **Figure 8.48**

back to the right this time, breathing out. Hold your breath out for a moment, staring at your thumb (Figure 8.49).

Repeat the sequence with your left foot forward.

T Pose (pictured, page 154)

Add the next three exercises between the Twisting Triangle and the Cat Breath (pages 33–34). When you are first learning this exercise, stand three to four feet from a chair or other support. Lean forward and hold on to the support with both hands. Lift your left leg in back as high as you can, ideally, parallel to the floor. Alternatively, brace yourself with both hands on the knee of your supporting leg. Keep your right (supporting) leg straight. Your torso and left leg should be in a straight line parallel to the floor. Keep your neck straight, breathe naturally, and look at a spot on the floor.

When you feel steady, release your grip on the support and place your palms together, pushing your arms out parallel to the floor. Relax your breath. Look forward at your hands. Lower your leg and return to a standing position. Rest until your breath returns to normal. Repeat on the opposite side.

Knee Bends

From the T Pose position, breathing naturally, keep your torso and lifted leg straight and parallel to the floor and, clasping your hands behind your back, gently bend your right knee and straighten (Figure 8.50). Try to do this without letting your shoulders and head bend toward the floor while your knee is bent. Keep breathing naturally. Stand up and rest. Repeat up to three times. Repeat on the opposite side.

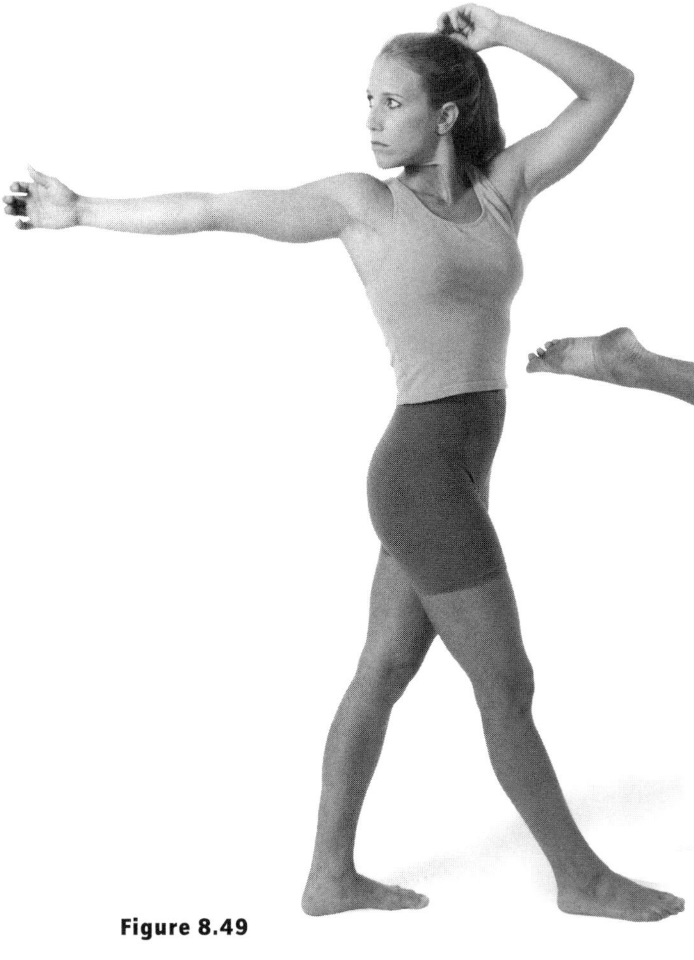

Figure 8.49

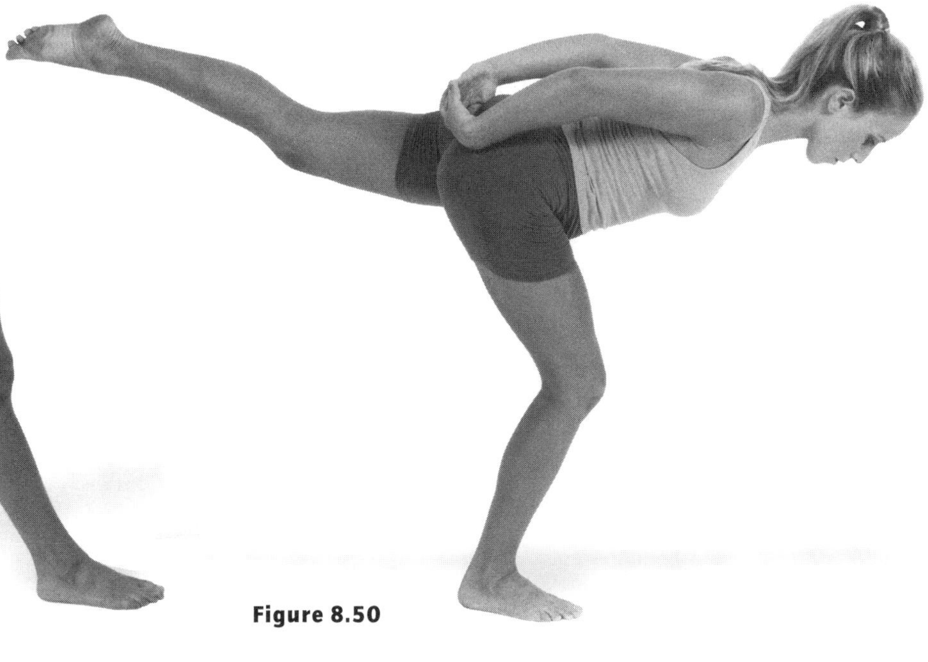

Figure 8.50

Warrior Pose (pictured, page 155)

When you are strong enough, you can perform this exercise immediately after the T Pose and Knee Bend on one side, then repeat the T Pose, Knee Bend, and Warrior on the opposite side.

Place both hands on your right knee and lift your left leg straight in back. Bend your right knee and let your torso rest on your right thigh as you slide your hands down to support either side of your right ankle. Keep your left leg high in back. Tuck your head. Breathe out and hold your breath out for a moment. Breathe in, slowly release, and repeat on the opposite side.

Variation: lace your fingers behind your back. If you can, lock your elbows, squeezing your shoulder blades together. Lift one leg as high as possible, bend your supporting leg, rest your chest on your thigh if possible, and lift your arms away from your back. Breathe out and hold for a moment. Release and switch sides.

Camel Pose (pictured, page 151)

Add the next two exercises between the Baby Pose and the Cobra Pose (pages 34–35). From a kneeling position, separate your knees slightly, arch your back and grasp your left heel with your left hand. Breathe normally. Do this once on each side to warm up. Then reach back and grasp both heels. Push your hips forward as far as possible without straining. Let your head gently fall back as you breathe out (unless you have a disk problem in your upper back or neck, in which case keep your head up).

Variation: if you are unable to grasp both heels at once, do the exercise once on each side in the beginning position instead.

Diamond Pose

Sit with the soles of your feet together, knees relaxed outward, hands clasped around your toes (Figure 8.51). Breathe in and straighten your back, then breathe out and bend forward, bringing your head toward your feet and letting your elbows fall outside your knees (Figure 8.52). Tuck your chin into your throat, contract your rectal muscles, and hold your breath out for a moment. Breathe in and release. Repeat twice more.

To limber your hips and knees, grasp your ankles instead of your feet and, when you breathe out and bend forward, press down on your thighs with your elbows (Figure 8.53).

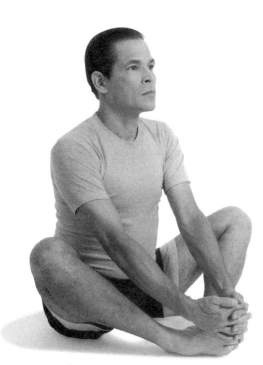

Figure 8.51

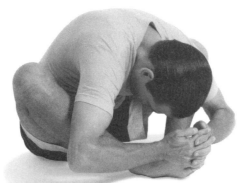

Figure 8.52

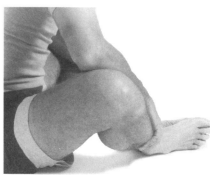

Figure 8.53

Boat Pose

Add this exercise between the Cobra Pose and the Knee Squeeze (pages 35–36). Lying on your stomach, stretch your arms on the floor over your head and place your forehead on the floor (Figure 8.54). Breathe out. Breathe in as you lift your arms, legs, and head, looking up through your forehead (Figure 8.55). Hold your breath in for a moment. Breathe out and release, bringing your arms and forehead back to the floor. Repeat twice more.

Plow Pose (pictured, pages 152–153)

Add this exercise after the Knee Squeeze (page 36). From a seated position, bend your knees and roll back and forth once or twice. Then roll back onto your shoulders, bringing your knees to your forehead and supporting your back with your hands. Breathe in, hold a moment, then breathe out, extending your legs behind your head, carefully trying to touch your toes to the floor. Breathe naturally and hold the position for several seconds.

If you wish, try this variation: straighten your arms on the floor over your head and hold for several seconds.

Breathe in and bend your knees back to your forehead, supporting your back with your hands, then roll forward to a cross-legged position, stretching your head and arms foward. Breathe naturally as you rest for about 10 seconds.

Note: if you have a disk problem in your neck or upper back, do not do this exercise; substitute the Easy Bridge (pages 163–164).

Sailing

Practice an all-around flexibility and strengthening routine, concentrating on the spine, to improve coordination, upper-body strength, and reaction time.

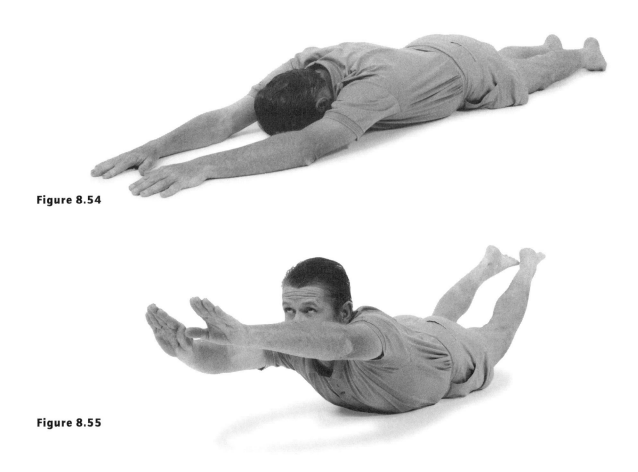

Figure 8.54

Figure 8.55

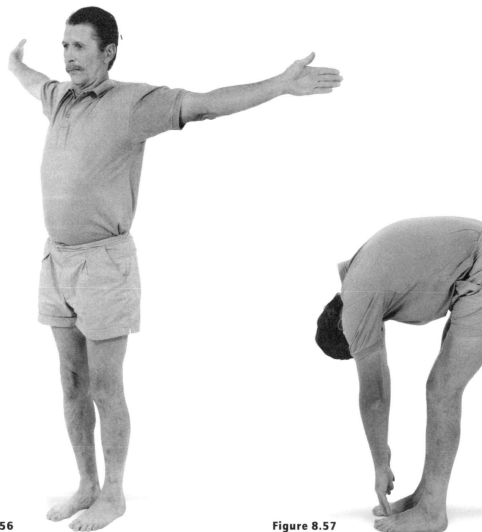

Figure 8.56

Figure 8.57

Practice breathing, relaxation, and meditation techniques at least once a day for steadiness and the opening of the intuitive voice.

Sailors often experience strains and muscle pulls due to extreme work by the upper body. The best way to prevent these injuries is through flexibility exercises and training in complete relaxation.

Modify your core routine as follows:

Full Bend

Add this exercise between the Neck Stretches and the Standing Sun Pose (pages 30–32). Stand with feet parallel, a few inches apart. Breathe out completely. Breathe in as you slowly raise your arms up and out to your sides, parallel to the floor (Figure 8.56).

Stretch back a little as you hold your breath in for a moment, then breathe out as you slowly bend forward, leading with your hands, until you are as far forward as possible. Let your whole body go limp (Figure 8.57). Now breathe in and slowly come back up, bringing your arms out to the sides again. Continue breathing in as you straighten up and out as you bend forward, matching your breath to your movement. Repeat several times.

Bow Variation (pictured, page 146)

Add this exercise between the Cat Breath and the Cobra V-Raise (page 34). Start on your hands and knees. Reach back with your left hand and grasp your right foot. Stare at one spot on the wall or floor for balance as you breathe in and lift your foot up and away from your body as far as possible. Hold your breath in for a moment. Breathe out, release slowly, and switch sides. Repeat three times on each side.

Plank Pose (pictured, page 157)

Add this exercise between the Cobra V-Raise and the Baby Pose (pages 34–35). From a hands-and-knees position, straighten your legs out behind you, supporting yourself on your hands. Raise your hips and lower your shoulders until your body is in a straight line supported on your hands and feet. Shift your weight to your right arm and breathe in as you lift your left arm straight in front of you. Focus your gaze on your outstretched hand. Hold your breath in for a moment. Breathe out and release.

Still supporting yourself on your right arm, breathe in as you bring your left arm to the side and up toward the ceiling. This will twist your body to the left as well. Look up toward your hand. Hold your breath in for a moment. Breathe out, bring your left hand down to the floor, and repeat the sequence on the opposite side. Then rest lying on your stomach.

Diamond Pose (pictured, page 160)

Add the next two exercises between the Baby Pose and the Cobra Pose (pages 34–35). Sit with the soles of your feet together, knees relaxed outward, hands clasped around your toes. Breathe in and straighten your back, then breathe out and bend forward, bringing your head toward your feet and letting your elbows fall outside your knees. Tuck your chin into your throat, contract your rectal muscles, and hold your breath out for a moment. Breathe in and release. Repeat twice more.

To limber your hips and knees, grasp your ankles instead of your feet and, when you breathe out and bend forward, press down on your thighs with your elbows.

Side Stretch

Sit up in a comfortable cross-legged position. Breathe in, then breathe out as you lean to the right and stretch your left arm up over your head and toward the right, stretching the entire left side of your torso (Figure 8.58). Hold your breath out for a moment. Breathe in as you release, then repeat on the opposite side.

Easy Bridge

Add the next two exercises between the Cobra Pose and the Knee Squeeze (pages 35–36). Lying on your back, bend your knees and separate your legs and feet several inches; place your arms at your sides, palms down (Figure 8.59). Breathe in, then breathe

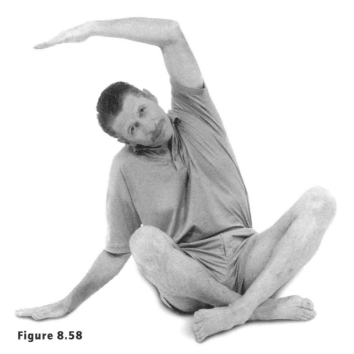

Figure 8.58

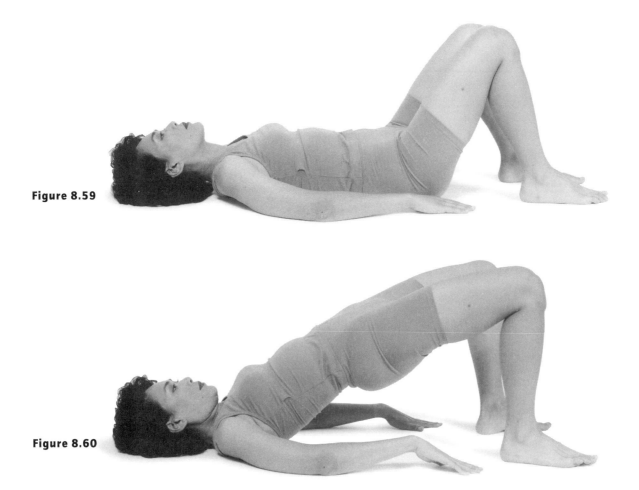

Figure 8.59

Figure 8.60

out as you lift your hips, arching your back and tucking your chin into your chest (Figure 8.60). Hold your breath out for a moment. Repeat twice more.

Variation: if you are very limber, you can grasp your ankles with both hands.

Shoulder Stand (pictured, pages 148–149)
In a seated position with your knees bent and your arms around your knees, roll back and forth a few times, then roll back onto your shoulders, immediately supporting your back with your hands and keeping your knees bent and touching your forehead.

Slowly straighten your legs toward the ceiling and push your back straighter by using your hands. Stare at the spot between your big toes and breathe out. Hold your breath out for a moment. Breathe in and relax your breath.

Bend your knees back to your forehead, supporting your back with your hands, then roll forward into a cross-legged position, reaching your head and arms forward. Breathe naturally as you rest for at least 10 seconds.

9

TEAM SPORTS

It's almost like instinct carries over more than just physical ability; to be able to read a pitch and then react to the pitch as a catcher or a player.

At times, to me as a catcher, when I am working with a pitcher and I'm putting down signs and he's not shaking, it's like we two are on the same page, the same wavelength. And I'm connecting through on his strengths to the hitter's weaknesses, and we're kind of dominating the game. I think that's kind of a subconscious feel where I'm thinking ahead without communicating with him but yet we're right in sync. And that's a pretty good high for a catcher or a pitcher to be in sync like that over the course of a year.

— TOMMY THOMPSON

It is the hardest thing to realize that you have just lost a game by one point, a game in which you played your heart out. As an athlete you put so much blood, sweat, and tears into everything that you do in order to achieve greatness for yourself and for your team. I remember how hard it was for me to realize that my basketball season was over this year. After the game, we all went out to dinner and I was the only one who was crying. I don't know what it was, maybe just the fact that it was over for the year, that I worked so hard on the court and off the court to be allowed to play again this year, to just see my team go out with not so much as a flicker broke my heart. A true athlete takes everything to heart and constantly thinks about the game and about what they could do better to help their team.

— EVE KENNEDY

When you practice Yoga techniques, you begin to direct attention to your inner body to such an extent that it would seem to be a detriment to your involvement in team sport. It is here that we can expand the old adage "It takes two halves to make a whole" to say that in reference to a team, all the separate blocks of a team go together to make a whole. The intense perfection of each block, or individual on the team, combines into a working pattern for the whole.

The ability to be a productive part of a team can depend on many things, but most precisely it depends on the intuitive ability of each player to know what the other players are doing and going to do, both on your own team and the opposite team. Great athletes have a natural intuitive feeling about the game that gives them the extra power of readiness for the unexpected. This extraordinary extra-intuitive sense can be learned and encouraged by daily practice of Yogic techniques.

Naturally, the preparation of the physical body is an important factor; however, I believe that the training of a team athlete is only complete when the inner quality of intuitive awareness balances the physical. Oftentimes, the team's intense attention to physical preparation becomes such a powerful demand that it seems to neglect the emotional, intuitive nature. Personal feelings are also part of the nature of the inner emotional/spiritual/power body.

In order to be a top-class team player, you need to know how the rest of your team feels as well as how you yourself feel. With this awareness, you can actually experience the other players' feelings in yourself while the game is in progress. This primitive awareness lies in everyone and usually shows itself in moments of extreme emotion such as fear or love. However, those athletes who use Yoga asans, breathing, and meditation techniques combined with the everyday physical training that is needed for a star-class athlete find that this awareness can appear on demand. I do not know if the great Bill Russell ever practiced Yoga, but he describes the experience I am talking about in this way:

> Every so often a Celtic game would heat up so that it became more than a physical or even mental game, and would be magical. That feeling is difficult to describe, and I certainly never talked about it when I was playing. When it happened I could feel my play rise to a new level . . . . At that special level all sorts of odd things happened . . . . It was almost as if we were playing in slow motion. During those spells I could almost sense how the next play would develop and where the next shot would be taken. Even before the other team brought the ball in bounds, I could feel it so keenly that I'd want to shout to my teammates, "It's coming there!"—except that I knew everything would change if I did. My premonitions would consistently be correct, and I always felt then that I not only knew all the Celtics by heart but also all the opposing players, and that they all knew me. There have been many times in my career when I felt moved or joyful, but these were the moments when I had chills pulsing up and down my spine.

The ideal routine to invite this innate sensitivity to emerge is at least 30 minutes of breathing, meditation, and asans immediately following your regular physical workout. This will have the effect of soothing and comforting the harsh demands of your physical workout. Your body is tired then and, because of the strenuous workout, slightly off guard. This makes it easy to move on to the Yogic routine without any preconceived notions of what it is supposed to be or do. You will find that your body will look forward to the time allotted because of the extremely pleasant feeling it gives you, and you will find very soon that the Yogic routine becomes as important to you as regular physical training. When you finish training, you will feel balanced and happy.

Yogic training works as a safe cooling-off period, allowing emotional reentry into nonphysical training time. In reality, of course, all time is training time for serious athletes. The goal of adequate training is never removed from the mind. This problem is difficult to communicate to others. For this reason it is especially necessary for you to learn how to relieve the pressure on your physical body in order to learn to call on the support of your emotional/spiritual/power body, eventually bringing the balance needed to use them together for the ultimate effort in strength. As you begin this practice, you will notice when your attention shifts from the physical to the

RECOVERY TIME

After all-out competition, and even after a hard training workout, muscle glycogen is badly depleted, and even with a high-carbohydrate diet, 48 hours is usually required for glycogen stores to recover. The recovery time is lengthened further if the muscles are not rested. Rest completely or have just a light workout on the day after all-out exertion, eat a high-carbohydrate diet, and come back strong!

emotional, but after a short time that switch of support strength will become effortless and automatic as one body or the other begins functioning when needed as balanced parts of the whole.

Many times the severe training of an athlete denies the emotional/spiritual/power body, ruthlessly relying on will to govern the physical. The inner body will endure this denial for only a short time; then it usually flares up, demanding attention. This is when athletes are likely to break out of training into destructive behavior that sometimes undermines the whole effort of their physical training. They sometimes use drugs, alcohol, and wild binges of any sort for relief from the denial of the inner body. These binges are usually precipitated by the need of the inner body to express itself. The emotional body shows its need, but binge relief is destructive to the physical body, the athlete, and, of course, the team. To be at your best as an athlete, you have to feel good about yourself. You can encourage this feeling by giving attention to the emotional/spiritual/power body that is not destructive.

To be the best in your ability as a team member, or indeed in any athletic training you choose, I suggest that you move slowly from the deep emotional awareness of meditation to ordinary physical consciousness. This will allow you to retain and incorporate the support value of the emotional/spiritual/power body into your normal physical awareness. Becoming aware of this subtle support will soon show you that what seemed to be two distinct, separate parts of your personality can now function as

one. Positioning the inner body and physical body in balance mends separateness in yourself; when this happens, all your strength as a whole person can be applied to your sport.

One of the things that I liked most about soccer that's unique, except maybe for hockey, is that all the players are equal. It's a total rhythm really. A good soccer team has a rhythm with all 10 players moving and in constant communication—often nonverbally, just a flow of play, like a school of fish. In soccer you definitely have to submerge your individual self to this team flow. The feeling of having a team flow is sometimes more pleasurable than scoring. We never thought we had failed even if we hadn't scored.

—Artie Guerin

Practice at least three asans, three breath exercises, and five minutes of meditation together in daily training. You will soon develop an intense intuitive emotional bonding that will enable you and your team to play as one person. This produces a powerful product in a team. The seemingly diverse physical and emotional qualities of all the players become channeled into one force, easily working together in harmony of effort. The German philosopher Hans-Georg Gadamer describes how, in what he calls "deep play," individual players lose their separateness from the full field of the game's action and begin to see themselves as part of a larger picture. One of the athletes we interviewed for this book, Alice Kennedy, described the experience perfectly:

A team is like a well-oiled machine. When all the gears are clicking together and every component is doing its part and we work as one to complete our task, it is the best feeling on earth. When we click it makes everyone happy. Individually I know that I don't want to let my teammates down, but I know that if I start to falter they will be there to pick me up. We act as one. We laugh together, cry together, win together, lose together, and achieve our team goals together. We often talk about team performance. A well-oiled machine can't run without individual parts such as gaskets, gears, and clamps. Each part plays an integral part in the performance of the machine. That is how a team is. Practice is like being "in the shop" where a gasket might have to be changed or the gears oiled. We all have individual roles that must be played for everything to work. And when it does, it is awesome. We become that well-oiled machine.

I encourage you to talk about the results of your emotional/spiritual/power body practice together as a team and with your coach. This will help heal the need for destructive emotional binges. If you watch carefully, you can always tell when an attack is coming. You can replace destructive behavior and soothe and feed your emotional body with the constructive, supportive techniques of breathing and meditation and the healing protective body movements of asans. The physical body will then feel protected against loss.

This brings up my last and most important point with regard to training for team sport. "Sacrifice for the good of the team" and "What happens to me personally is not important, the important thing here is team success" are common statements that are often heard in team training. However, the athlete who joins a team may feel a loss of personal achievement. Individual athletes always feel strongly about their own performance and are able to sacrifice the power of the performance to the team only if they are able to draw on the inner strength of the emotional/spiritual/power body. Yogic discipline allows them to withstand the sacrifice without emotional loss. Research has shown that there is a specific primitive quality in the brain that enjoys team involvement. If an athlete can be part of a team without feeling loss, real enjoyment is there.

Many times fine athletes will be unable to work with a team without feeling, and creating, constant upset. If they are fortunate, usually after many arduous, eroding transfers from one team to another, they are able to find other team players and a coach that they can be comfortable with; only then can they begin to show their ability in its highest form. This clearly shows that their performance needs the support of the emotional/spiritual/power body. Some-

It is absolutely awesome to watch one of my teams playing together as one unit. It is also awesome to be one of the team members out there on the court or field making things happen. The best feeling is when you play as a team for the entire game. That happened this year during my lacrosse season. We played a team that was nationally ranked in the NCAAs and we played so amazingly, everyone felt like they had a part in it, even the people on the bench who never got to play. After the game, we all talked about it, about how wonderful it felt, and about how we knew that we had it in ourselves to give 100 percent each.

—Eve Kennedy

times athletes will find an ingenious coach who recognizes the problem of fear of loss individual athletes can experience when they become part of a group, but it may take a long time.

It is a sacrifice to give up your personal physical ego to a team. In order to do it happily, you need to have full confidence in your inner emotional strength and ability. In other words, you feel no loss; you know that a limitless supply of power is available to you from within yourself.

I am a big football fan, and I really enjoy watching some of the great stars of the sport who are able to bring all their power to the game without demanding or receiving extra attention for their services. This is a representation of true greatness in sport. Whether they handle the ball 2 times or 20 times, their ability for top performance remains the same. Because of physical and emotional balance, they bring power to the game to be used when the team needs it, not when the player thinks it should be used. They rarely complain that there was no chance to show their ability. The enjoyment of knowing that the powerful ability is theirs to use at any time replaces their personal ego-loss to the team effort. This outlook allows the diverse factions of the team to pull together as one body, resulting in great performance and ability.

For best results, practice together with your coaches and also at home once or twice a day when you are alone. If the suggested routine is too long,

THE PRE-GAME MEAL

Food Myth: the pre-event meal of steak and eggs guarantees top performance.

"It's really the opposite of when I was in college playing soccer. They used to feed us training meals of steak and potatoes; I guess when you're twenty years old you can get away with a lot of things."

—Artie Guerin

Protein and fat slow stomach emptying and do not help build glycogen stores needed during exercise, so the ideal pregame meal is a low-fat, low-protein meal with a high starch content, such as pasta, cereal, or pancakes, eaten two to four hours before competition. This allows time for the body to digest and absorb the food and transform it into glycogen. Small amounts of carbohydrate foods or drinks may be consumed shortly before competing without affecting performance.

begin with three asans, done in a room alone and in silence, with concentrated attention to your physical body. Then practice three to five minutes of the Complete Breath, described on page 20, ending with 15 to 20 minutes of meditation. Review the precautions for protecting yourself from noise and staying warm that are discussed in Chapter 2. Do not practice with pets in the room. Be careful not to leap out of your meditation practice; give yourself a few minutes of quiet reentry into normal activity.

The results of regular practice can be seen in as little as a week. Communication with your team will come easily, and because of that, you will save a lot of time in practice. Practice routines will lose their boring quality and will become exciting and profitable.

The Sport Routine for Teams

Alter your core routine as follows:

Elbow Touch
Add this exercise between the Elbow Twist and the Arm Circles (pages 29–30). Place your fingers on your shoulders, elbows out to the sides. Breathing normally, move your elbows toward each other in front (Figure 9.1), then squeeze them toward each other in back (Figure 9.2), keeping them at the same level. Repeat several times.

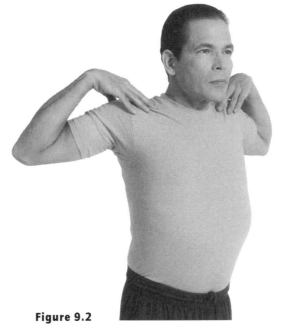

Figure 9.1   **Figure 9.2**

Full Bend Variation

Add this exercise between the Neck Stretches and the Standing Sun Pose (pages 30–32). Stand with feet parallel. Clasp your hands behind your back. If you can, press your palms together. For an even greater stretch, lock your elbows so your shoulder blades are squeezed together. Breathe in and lift your arms in back as far as you can without straining (Figure 9.3). Breathe out and bend forward, tucking your chin and keeping your arms in position (Figure 9.4). Hold your breath out for a moment. Breathe in and straighten. Repeat the exercise twice more.

T Pose

Add the next two exercises between the Standing Sun Pose and the Hip Rotation (pages 31–32). When you are first learning this exercise, stand three to four feet from a chair or other support. Lean forward and hold on to the support with both hands. Lift your left leg in back as high as you can (Figure 9.5), ideally, parallel to the floor. Alternatively, brace both hands on the knee of your supporting leg (Figure 9.6). Keep your right (supporting) leg straight. Your torso and left leg should

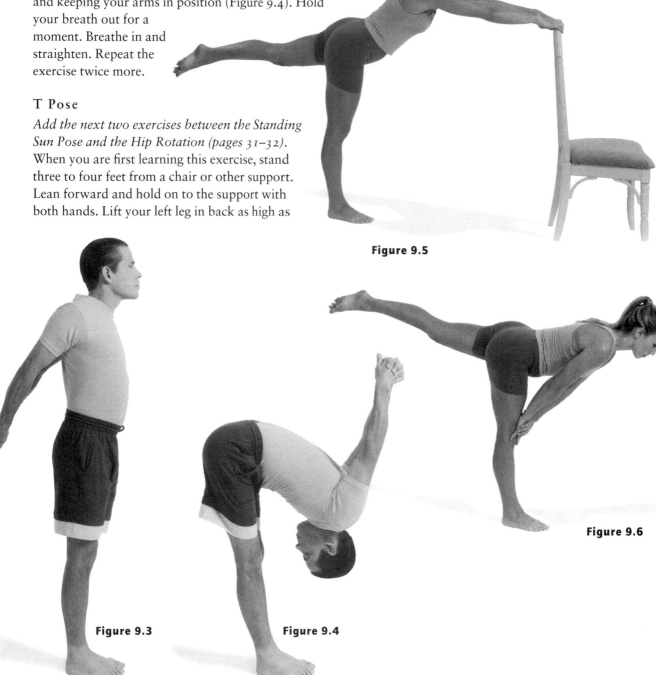

Figure 9.5

Figure 9.3

Figure 9.4

Figure 9.6

be in a straight line parallel to the floor. Keep your neck straight, breathe naturally, and look at a spot on the floor.

When you feel steady, release your grip on the support and place your palms together, pushing your arms out parallel to the floor (Figure 9.7). Relax your breath. Look forward at your hands. Lower your leg and return to a standing position. Rest until your breath returns to normal. Repeat on the opposite side.

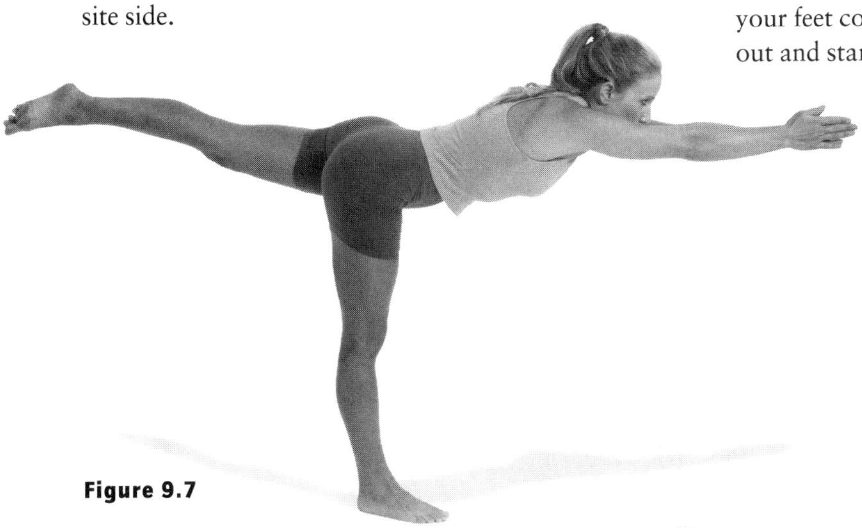

Figure 9.7

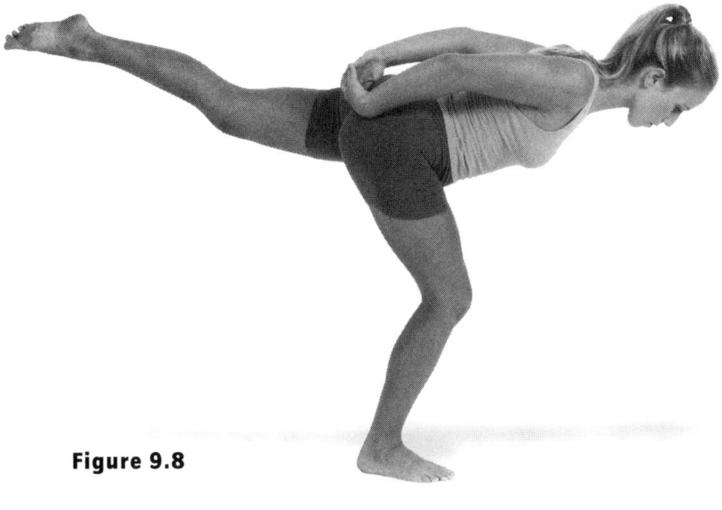

Figure 9.8

Knee Bends

From the T Pose position, breathing naturally, keep your torso and lifted leg straight and parallel to the floor and, clasping your hands behind your back, gently bend your right knee and straighten (Figure 9.8). Try to do this without letting your shoulders and head bend toward the floor while your knee is bent. Keep breathing naturally. Stand up and rest. Repeat up to three times. Repeat on the opposite side.

Crow Pose

Add this exercise between the Cat Breath and the Cobra V-Raise (page 34). Squat on your toes, separate your knees, and place your hands on the floor between your knees about a foot apart. Bend your elbows and place the inside joint of your knees on your elbows (Figure 9.9; you'll have to lift your hips slightly to do this). Carefully lean forward, resting your bent knees on the back of your elbows, until your feet come off the floor (Figure 9.10). Breathe out and stare at one spot on the floor. Hold your breath out for a moment. Relax and rest.

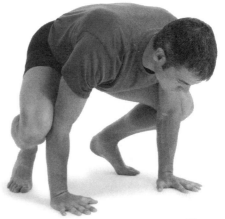

Figure 9.9

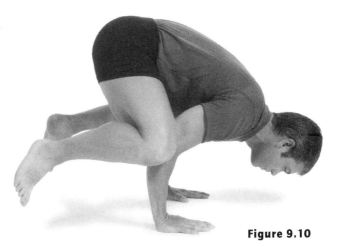

Figure 9.10

Lunge Series

Add this exercise between the Cobra V-Raise and the Baby Pose (pages 34–35). With your toes pointed inward, spread your legs as far apart as you comfortably can. Breathe in as you turn completely toward the left and bend your left leg, bringing your left elbow underneath your left knee and resting on both fists (Figure 9.11). Keep your right leg straight if you can; if that position is too strenuous, rest your knee on the floor. Bend your head toward the floor as you breathe out. Hold your breath out for a moment. Breathe in and release. Repeat on the opposite side.

Breathe in as you turn back to the left. Breathe out as you rest both elbows on the floor with your left elbow inside your left knee, lower your right knee to the floor, clasp your hands, and bend your head toward your hands (Figure 9.12). Hold your breath out for a moment.

Breathe in as you push yourself up, rest your left arm on your left thigh, and straighten your right arm and your right leg (Figure 9.13). Breathe out and hold your breath out for a moment.

Breathe in and release. With your legs in the same position, breathe out as you stretch both arms out to the sides, resting your chest on your left thigh (Figure 9.14). Hold your breath out for a moment.

Bring your left hand to the floor on the inside of your left leg. Breathe in and stretch your right arm straight up toward the ceiling (Figure 9.15). Look at your outstretched fingers and hold your breath in for a moment.

Breathe out, bring your arm down, swivel over to the right, and repeat the series facing right.

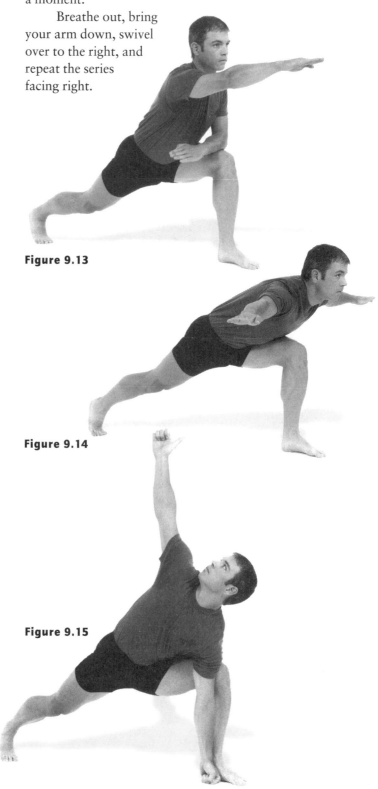

Figure 9.13

Figure 9.14

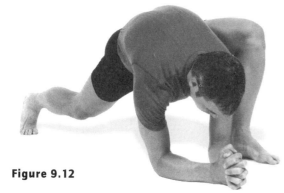

Figure 9.11

Figure 9.12

Figure 9.15

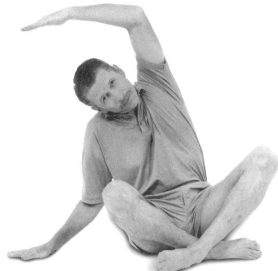

Figure 9.16

Side Stretch

Add the next four exercises between the Baby Pose and the Cobra Pose (pages 34–35). Sit up in a comfortable cross-legged position. Breathe in, then breathe out as you

lean to the right and stretch your left arm up over your head and toward the right, stretching the entire left side of your torso (Figure 9.16). Hold your breath out for a moment. Breathe in as you release, then repeat on the opposite side.

Seated Sun Pose

Bring both legs straight out in front of you and flex your toes. Sit straight, breathe out with your arms at your sides (Figure 9.17), then breathe in as you raise your arms in a wide circle to the sides (Figure 9.18) and overhead. Press your palms together, look up, visualize the sun, and stretch from the rib cage (Figure 9.19). Hold your breath in for a moment.

Breathe out as you bend forward, tucking your chin toward your chest. Grasp your ankles, bend your elbows, and pull your torso toward your legs (remember to pull by bending your arms, not by pushing with your lower back). Hold your breath out for a moment.

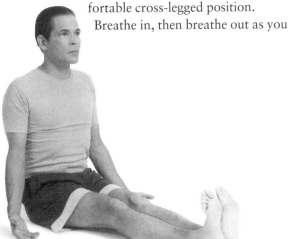

Figure 9.17

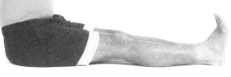

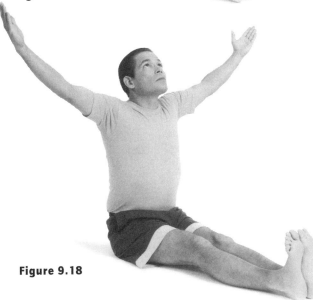

Figure 9.18

Figure 9.19

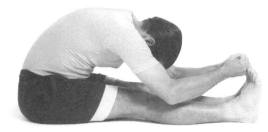

Figure 9.20

If you are limber enough to reach your feet (and still bend your elbows), grasp your big toes as shown (Figures 9.20 and 9.21).

Release and breathe in, bringing your arms to the sides and over your head again. Stretch and look up as before. Breathe out and bring your arms back down to your sides. Repeat three times.

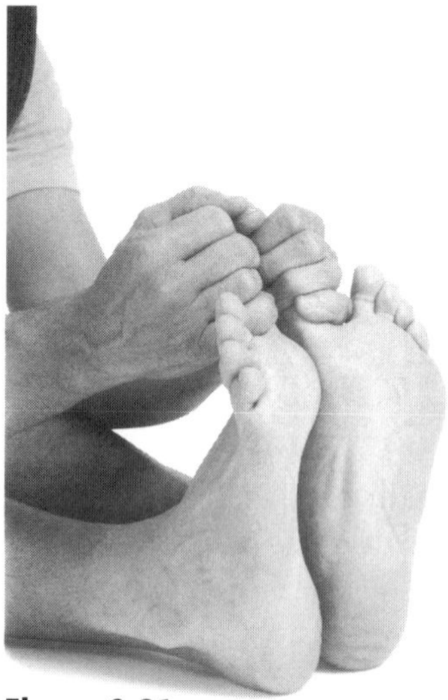

Tortoise Pose

Straighten your legs and separate them as far as possible. Straighten your back and breathe in as you raise your arms in a wide circle to the sides and over your head (Figure 9.22). Breathe out as you bend forward, reaching down over your right leg. Grasp your calf, ankle, or foot with both hands (Figure 9.23). If you can reach your toes easily, grasp the big toe as in the Alternate Seated Sun Pose (see page 143). Hold your breath out for a moment. Breathe in and raise your arms back over your head, then breathe out and lower your arms to your sides. Repeat three times to each side, then do the exercise three times reaching for both feet (Figure 9.24).

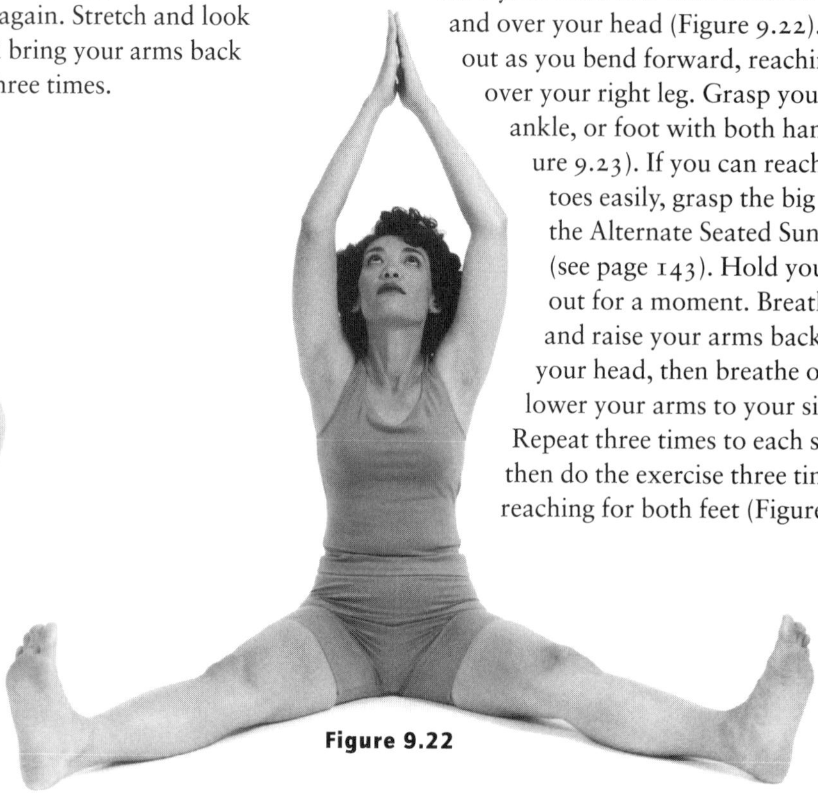

Figure 9.21

Figure 9.22

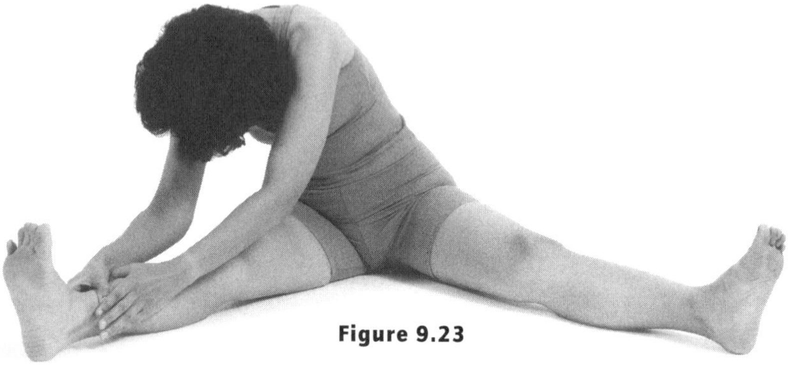

Figure 9.23

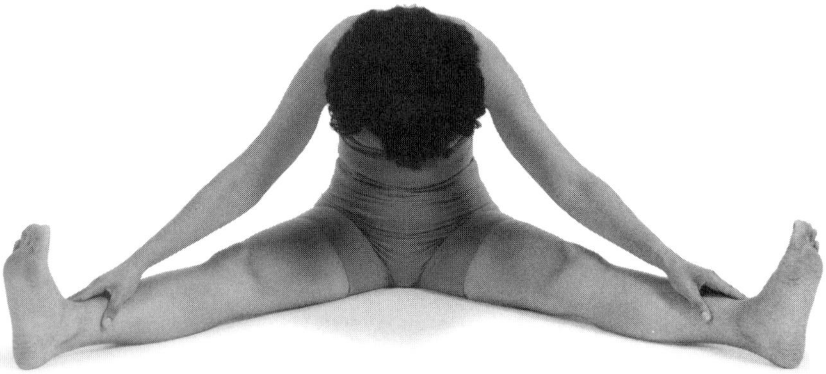

Figure 9.24

Diamond Pose

Sit with the soles of your feet together, knees relaxed outward, hands clasped around your toes (Figure 9.25). Breathe in and straighten your back, then breathe out and bend forward, bringing your head toward your feet and letting your elbows fall outside your knees (Figure 9.26). Tuck your chin into your throat, contract your rectal muscles, and hold your breath out for a moment. Breathe in and release. Repeat twice more.

To limber your hips and knees, grasp your ankles instead of your feet and, when you breathe out and bend forward, press down on your thighs with your elbows (Figure 9.27).

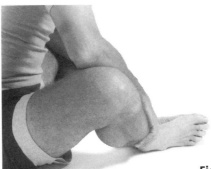

Figure 9.27

Back Strengthener Series

Add these exercises between the Cobra Pose and the Knee Squeeze (pages 35–36). Stretch your arms on the floor over your head and place your forehead on the floor (Figure 9.28). Breathe out. Breathe in as you lift your arms, legs, and head, looking up through your forehead (Figure 9.29; this exercise is also called the Boat Pose). Hold your breath in for a moment.

Breathe out and release, bringing both arms straight out to the sides, palms down, and forehead to the floor (Figure 9.30). Rest a moment, then

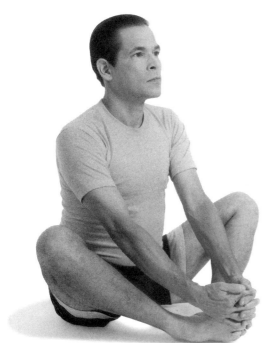

Figure 9.25

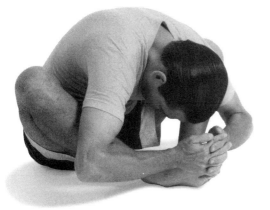

Figure 9.26

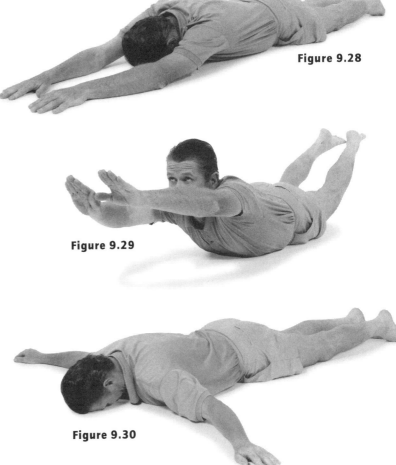

Figure 9.28

Figure 9.29

Figure 9.30

breathe in as you lift your arms, legs, and head, looking up through your forehead (Figure 9.31). Hold your breath in for a moment.

Breathe out and release, bringing your arms down to your sides (Figure 9.32). Rest a moment, then breathe in as you lift your arms, legs, and head, looking up through your forehead (Figure 9.33). Hold your breath in for a moment.

Breathe out and release, bringing your arms behind your back with your fingers clasped (Figure 9.34). Rest a moment, then breathe in as you lift your arms, legs, and head, pressing your palms together and straightening your arms as much as possible so your shoulder blades are squeezed together and your arms stretch away from your body (Figure 9.35). Look up through your forehead. Hold your breath in for a moment.

Breathe out and release, bending your knees and grasping your feet with both hands (Figure 9.36). Rest a moment with your forehead to the floor, then breathe in as you lift, pulling up on your feet so you balance on your stomach (Figure 9.37; this position is also called the Bow Pose). Look up through your forehead. Hold your breath in for a moment. Breathe out and release. Rest on your stomach.

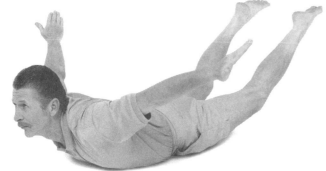

Figure 9.31

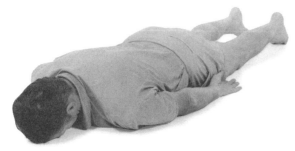

Figure 9.32

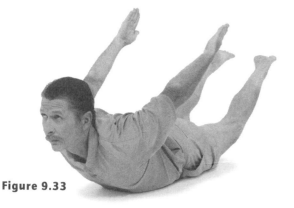

Figure 9.33

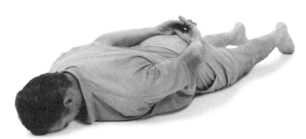

Figure 9.34

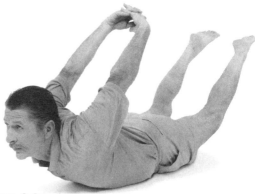

Figure 9.35

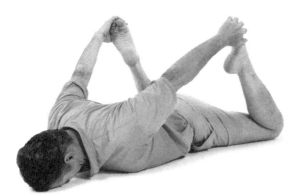

Figure 9.36

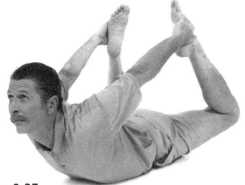

Figure 9.37

Easy Bridge and Wheel

Add this exercise after the Knee Squeeze (page 36).
Lying on your back, bend your knees and separate
your legs and feet several inches; place your arms at
your sides, palms down (Figure 9.38). Breathe in,
then breathe out as you lift your hips, arching your
back and tucking your chin into your chest (Figure
9.39). Hold your breath out for a moment. Repeat
twice more.

Variation: if you are very limber, you can grasp
your ankles with both hands.

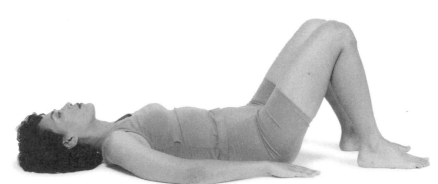

*I used to play a lot of team sports and when I
started with triathlons I missed the interactions
with teammates. Last year I did an adventure
race, which is an event where you have three- or
four-person teams depending on the event. You
must start as a team and finish as a team. The
race involves orienteering, canoeing, mountain
biking, running, and obstacle courses. This
style of racing has filled a void I felt with
triathlons and has proved to be a great cross-
training tool.*

—Dale O'Hara

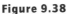

Figure 9.38

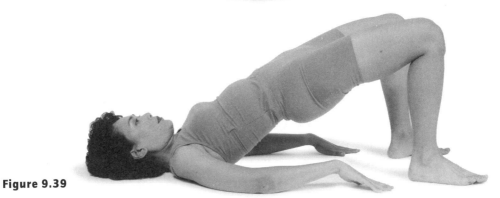

Figure 9.39

If you are strong enough, try the Wheel: place your hands next to your head, fingers pointing toward your feet (Figure 9.40). Breathe in and push up so you are resting on your head (Figure 9.41). If you can, continue pushing up into the full position (Figure 9.42). Hold your breath in for a moment.

Breathe out and lower your body to the floor, straighten your legs, bring your arms down to your sides, and rest.

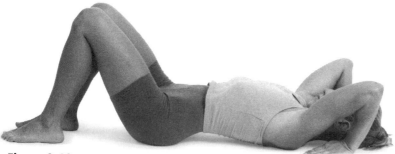

Figure 9.40

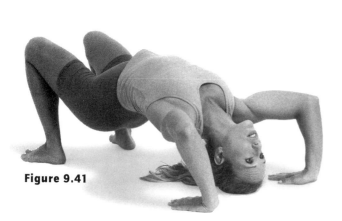

Figure 9.41

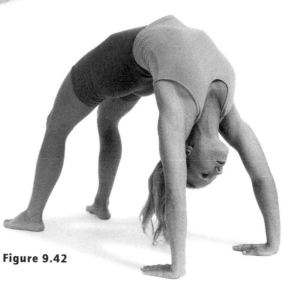

Figure 9.42

10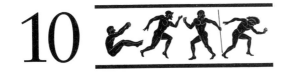

SOME THOUGHTS FOR THE COACH

You have to model not being selfish, not being self-centered yourself. I show the kids on the court that I'll play somebody not just to win. I'll play a kid who gives me a hundred percent and I'll let the superstar sit down if he has a bad attitude or is not team oriented. You have to show it. You can't just talk it. You talk it a lot, though, because most of it's verbal. You just continually talk it, and hopefully you plant a seed and the kids will see what it's about. You just have to see those teachable moments and jump at them when you see them.

Helping the guys develop self-confidence is the hardest part of the game today, because everything that they emulate on television is all really individual goals. It's all about "me." Team is the hardest thing to build.

I had a young man who had a problem with his weight, but he worked just as hard as another guy who is going to play division-one ball. He was right there with him. Now he didn't have the great skills, so he worked just as hard. And it made him our second-best player on the team this year. A guy who probably wouldn't have played for anybody four years ago because of his weight. He wouldn't have made that team. He worked hard on keeping his weight under control, and then he kept working on his skills, kept working hard. And he played a lot last year. I'm trying to get him into college somewhere. He's the kind of kid you don't mind working for. He'll go to college and he'll work hard. He won't play much but he'll work in his team. It's all about team. He knows what it takes and he knows his limitations, and he lives with those and works to be the best he can be.

—LEMUEL ANDREWS

No book on sports would be complete without a discussion of the role of the coach. A good coach is a friend, a parent-surrogate, and a thorn in your side as well as a trainer. In order to coach most effectively, the coach must have been a player, but more importantly, he or she must have the ability to translate the playing experience to others.

The communication between coach and athlete is not always verbal. In fact, the best communication often is unspoken; it rises from the unlimited source of intuition, which is available to all of us but is rarely recognized or welcomed. Probably this is because intuition is seen as something unreliable; like a hunch, it seems not to come when summoned, but rather, seemingly out of the blue.

> We don't want our football players to think during a game, because thinking takes too long. We want them to react—to have the correct moves so ingrained in practice that instinct guides them to the right place at the right time. It's like giving a speech; it's the drudge work and research you put into it beforehand that lets you make your points with freewheeling assurance.
>
> —Bill Parcells, *Finding a Way to Win*

Whether you are working with an individual athlete or with a team, the single most important quality needed to be a successful coach, as I see it, is a highly developed intuitive power. This gives you a hypersensitive awareness of the athletes in your care. You can then learn to rely on the unknown quality of intuition so that it becomes a practical tool at your disposal.

One of the best uses of intuition is in the often difficult task of molding a group of individual athletes into a team. Any team is, of course, made up of single athletes who join together in effort. The difficulty lies in the joining. The art of coaching is the blending of many diverse personalities into one powerful unit. To do this, coaching requires a remarkable ability to contact a depth within each member of that team so that they all function as one person, with one goal.

> The stuff that I did and coaches made me do when I was growing up, you can't get away with that today. Kids are a little more vocal and a little bit more liberal in their thinking and they don't want to hear that. They're not willing to put up with a lot of that. So you have to be a friend, not the big guy, the boss. That attitude they don't go for much. At least that's what I have noticed over the years. But on the other hand they still respect you. They know what you expect and they give you that. So I don't have a problem with that.
>
> —Lemuel Andrews

> Remember you've got to communicate always. Teach the game. It's an ongoing process. Even if the other team makes mistakes, you know that our team can learn from them.
>
> —Tommy Thompson

You can do this most efficiently by calling on your intuitive ability, which can be greatly increased by practicing meditation. Use this technique to find a solution to any team problem. For instance, if a member of your team has a great ability for the game but cannot get along with other team members, you can use meditation to call upon your intuition, which can give you the perfect solution to the problem.

Begin your meditation exercise by sitting silently for a few moments (see Chapter 2 for how to practice meditation). Then begin a conversation with yourself about the problem. Completely discuss the problem with yourself, and tell yourself you need a solution. Then become completely silent. Stop all conversation with yourself in your head. Simply refuse to speak, physically or mentally. Sit in perfect silence for two or three minutes and allow the request for the answer to the problem to sit in your mind unmoving.

You may find it very difficult at first to maintain silence in your mind, but eventually you will be able to achieve one or two minutes of quietness, and when that happens you will often realize a solution to the problem. You will notice an enhanced ability to communicate with the members of your team in a way that they can understand even though each one of them has a different outlook. This is because you will be able to communicate through the inner emotional/spiritual/power body, which is the same in all of us. The physical body is very different in everyone, but the emotional body is the same. Therefore, language developed with the emotional body can be clear and easily understood. The really important point here is that by functioning in this way, you will be able to get your ideas across to your team much more easily. This will save hours of time in training and help the team perform as a whole unit.

Meditative techniques can also be used by coaching staff to help athletes reenter the competitive arena from their everyday lives. Needless to say, a certain poise is needed to be able to switch from "normal" life into a full-fledged effort of performance. This is especially difficult when athletes have to travel, as when teams go on the road or when athletes have to travel to competitions. The best techniques for these stressful situations are breathing and meditation exercises practiced as a group. This can be done on a charter flight, on a bus, or in a hotel room upon arrival.

> Nutrition is really important. I do tell them what's good for them to play the sport. So we stay away from the sugars and the sweets. We try to tell them to stay away from sodas. It's hard for them. Carbonated drinks are there and there are fast foods and they jump at them. The ones that really want me to stay on them, they'll tell me, "Coach, when we stop, don't let me get this." I had a player who did that. "Don't let me get any pies. Just stand right there and make sure I don't get any pies." They're dedicated. They know that it's tough for them. It's hard for them to have that self-control. But I think nutrition is 50, 60 percent of the ball game out there for us. You have to eat right in order to play this game. Prior to playing a game I think you should take care of yourself.
>
> —Lemuel Andrews

Sit together in silence for a minute or two in any seated position in which the spine is straight (or lying flat on the floor), perform three Complete Breath exercises (see Chapter 2), then stop all inner conversation, and sit together in total silence for about five minutes. This will encourage the emotional nature to come forward in support of the physical bodies of the athletes and also the team. You then will have stopped the scattered, fragmented feeling that accompanies team or performance stress compounded by the stress of travel. This exercise produces a strong feeling of confidence and helps the team maintain a restful state in unfamiliar surroundings. Athletes or performers can then head into competition knowing that extra strength is there for them to use, resulting in peak individual performance in a team atmosphere.

> For team unity we get together away from the court, maybe get together at my house or other coaches' houses for cookouts, or go to games together. Because I don't like them to think about basketball all the time. We talk about life and work, school; the things that are important in their life. We may watch some games or something together, but we get away from the court and try to develop that off-court relationship.
>
> Some kids come to the team a little overweight, and some come in a little clumsy, no hands. Some come with no speed, no jumping ability. You have them all work on all of that. But then you emphasize certain things with certain players. You develop a workout plan for them. I work out with them to let them know I'll suffer some of the pain with them, and also to show them that they're not hurting as bad as they say they are. Some guys think I couldn't do what I ask them to do, so I just go out and show them that I still can do a little bit of it.
>
> —Lemuel Andrews

Coaches have a marvelous ability to enjoy all the emotional fireworks of athletic performance vicariously. They can experience all the thrill of an athlete's performance from the sidelines. Coaches are often subject to heavy mood swings because they cannot, as individuals, be involved in the expression of sport, but must instead teach and encourage others to do it. It is extremely difficult to explain an idea of motion or action unless you are doing the action as you explain it. Conversation becomes difficult, and because of this, the intuitive communication of a coach to athletes becomes paramount.

Obviously, when coaching a team sport, it is impossible to show in movement what an entire team has to do in a game. Coaches can develop a whole new way of communicating—one that is so appealing that they can constantly maintain the attention of the entire team. Steve Owens, former coach of the New York Giants, made a great point: "Coaching is like a monkey on a stick. You pass the same fellows on the way down as you do on the way up." And it is true. Coaches never can stay in one position. They cannot always produce a winning team. They are totally dependent on what they have to work with and how well they can communicate their knowledge of how to use this commodity. There is, therefore, a need for super-tolerance that grows in coaching—a tolerance of winning and losing and the difficult job of directing the athletes to best use the qualities that lie within them.

> I remember one time I was in a hitting slump in Durham, North Carolina. I was hitting about three hundred with the Durham Bulls and was zero for July. I didn't get a hit in like seventy-eight at-bats, and it dropped me down to about two-twenty-six. And the coach just came up to me and said, "Hey, you're not swinging the bat too bad. You're getting no results. Why don't you go up there and just simplify things, see the ball, try to hit the ball the other way. If that doesn't work, then bunt for a hit." And I got a couple of hits that night. Broke out of it. And it just was somebody simplifying things with me. I was putting more pressure on myself. He just simplified things: "See the ball, don't try to pull it. Work the other field. And just go up there with a plan and do it"—and it worked and I felt good about it.
>
> —Tommy Thompson

It takes a long time to build a winning team. Maintaining balance and emotional composure in losing and winning is extremely difficult. The coach feels his whole team's frustration and upset as well as his own. There is much talk about being a "good loser," but being a "good loser" takes tremendous self-confidence, and that confidence has to infect all athletes in the coach's care. Lemuel Andrews, the high school basketball coach we interviewed, talked about the most important quality he tries to instill in players:

> It's character. Knowing how to deal with the ups and downs. Not a lot of guys have the courage to face their weaknesses and try to be strong and to try to get stronger, try to build upon them. Being honest with yourself and being realistic about who you are and where you're going. And always questioning in yourself the honesty thing. "Let me see what's the real truth to it. Let me face the real facts here." Just build on the good; take the good as well as the bad and build on it.

George Brett, former third baseman for the Kansas City Royals, described loss as he experienced it: "Losing is like kissing your grandmother with her teeth out." Nobody wants to be a loser, but losing is the opposite of winning; without losing, there would be no way to measure winning. Losing is the balancing factor of sports, and maintaining balance is an essential discipline of coaching because of constant emotional drain. Emotional balance in winning is equally important.

> Like in any sport, you want the athletes to do well. When they do, you share their feeling of self-accomplishment. I know my athletes have achieved peak performance when everything they do in competition looks effortless. When the team is operating as a unit, we have a lot of team spirit. The athletes really seem to support each other—not only in their successes, but also when things are not going well. I try to instill the idea that everyone is important and everyone makes a contribution to the team.
>
> —Rick Dodson, gymnastics coach

In a majority of cases, coaches are still active athletes, and fortunately they have a good physical base to work from. Their athletic training in early years stands in good support for the later years of increased tension and stress. Adding a regular Yogic routine can provide the keystone for total support of the coaching program and can add years to the productivity of a coaching career. The addition of at least three asans, three breath exercises, and 15 to 30 minutes of meditation will bring on the balance that is needed in daily life. If coaches practice this Yogic discipline with single athletes or a team, an intense bonding will promote very clear communication with very few words.

Coaches' personal lives may suffer unless they pay attention to the need for constant connection with the inner emotional/spiritual/power body. By following a regular Yogic routine, coaches will be able to maintain secure family relationships while giving total support and attention to a single athlete or a team. If coaches ignore the connection to their inner body, as well as that of the team, they will find it impossible to be all things to all people. Coaches need extra nurturing that can only come from inside themselves.

The first appearance of the help that Yogic practice will provide is the ability to rest. Usually a coach's body is under such severe strain that even in rest periods, his or her mind repeats and works over the day's events. Meditation will allow the mind to step back from this constant internal conversation into healing silence. The heart, the head, the whole physical body heals as it rests.

Remarkably, it is this time of rest that allows a supersensitivity to emerge. Intuition blooms and serves to cut debilitating conversation time in half. Intuition provides information to you before it can be put into words. As intuitive power grows, the coach rests on a new support of self-confidence. Coaching seems to be a main target for criticism. Meditation practice will allow you to stand steady and confident in the storm of criticism that accompanies all sports, especially coaching. This needed protection will allow the coach to carry through ideas with less frustration and will supply the joy of seeing those ideas take shape in the athletes and the game.

The coach then becomes the ultimate archer, lifting the athlete, as the arrow, to the bow of support and training, to hit the perfect mark of shining excellence in sports.

RESOURCES ON THE SPORTS EXPERIENCE AND SPORTS NUTRITION

Playing in the Zone, Andrew Cooper. Boston: Shambhala Press, 1998.

In the Zone, Michael Murphy and Rhea A. White. New York: Penguin/Arkana, 1978, 1995.

Second Wind, Bill Russell and Taylor Branch. New York: Random House, 1979.

Finding a Way to Win, Bill Parcells. New York: Doubleday, 1995.

Sports Injury Handbook, Allan M. Levy and Mark L. Fuerst. New York: John Wiley and Sons, 1993.

The Sports Medicine Bible, Lyle J. Micheli. New York: Harper Perennial, 1995.

Tips on Avoiding, Living with, and Curing Tennis Elbow, Artie Guerin. Article available by sending check or money order for $4.95 to P.O. Box 20722, Sarasota, FL 34276.

The Ultimate Sports Nutrition Handbook, Ellen Coleman. Palo Alto, CA: Bull Publishing Co., 1996.

Championship Sports Psychology, Dr. Keith Bell. Austin, TX: Keel Publications, 1983.

Power Foods: High-Performance Nutrition for High-Performance People, Liz Applegate. Emmaus, PA: Rodale Press, 1994.

Nancy Clark's Sports Nutrition Guidebook, 2d ed., Nancy Clark. Champaign, IL: Human Kinetics, 1996.

Optimum Sports Nutrition, Dr. Michael Colgan. Ronkonkoma, NY: Advanced Research Press, 1993.

RESOURCES FROM THE AMERICAN YOGA ASSOCIATION

Further information on Yoga is available from the American Yoga Association. To obtain general information about Yoga, including a complete catalog and guidelines for choosing a qualified teacher, send a self-addressed envelope stamped with postage for two ounces to the following address:

American Yoga Association
P.O. Box 19986
Sarasota, FL 34276

For questions about Yoga, write to the address above, or contact us by telephone or E-mail:

Telephone: (941) 927-4977
Fax: (941) 921-9844
E-mail: Yogamerica@aol.com
Website: http://users.aol.com/amyogaassn

We offer classes in the Cleveland, Ohio, area. For more information, write or call:

American Yoga Association
P.O. Box 18105
Cleveland Hts., OH 44106
Telephone: (216) 556-1313

Books

The American Yoga Association Beginner's Manual. Complete instructions for more than 90 Yoga exercises and breathing techniques; three 10-week curriculum outlines; chapters on nutrition, philosophy, stress management, pregnancy; and more.

20-Minute Yoga Workouts: The Perfect Program for the Busy Person. Brief routines that anyone can fit into the busiest schedule. Includes chapters on women's issues, toning and shaping, the "20-minute challenge," and workouts to do while traveling.

The American Yoga Association's New Yoga Challenge. Routines for energy, strength, flexibility, focus, and stability offer more vigorous Yoga workouts for body and mind. The last chapter, "The Powerful Individual," teaches readers how to design their own routines.

The American Yoga Association Wellness Book. A basic routine to maintain health and well-being, plus chapters on how Yoga can specifically help with arthritis, heart disease, back pain, PMS and menopause, weight management, insomnia, headaches, and other health conditions.

Easy Does It Yoga. For those with physical limitations, this book includes instruction in specially adapted Yoga exercises that can be done in a chair or in bed, breathing techniques, and meditation.

The Easy Does It Yoga Trainer's Guide. A complete manual for how to begin teaching the Easy Does It Yoga program to adults with physical limitations due to age, convalescence, substance abuse, injury, or obesity. Excellent for health professionals, activities directors, physical therapists, home health aides, and others who work with the elderly or in rehabilitative services.

Meditation. A collection of excerpts from lectures and classes on the subject of meditation, including a section of questions and answers from students.

Reflections of Love. A collection of excerpts from Alice Christensen's lectures and classes on the subject of love.

The Light of Yoga. A chronicle of the unusual circumstances that catapulted Alice Christensen into Yoga practice in the early 1950s, including the teachers and experiences that shaped her first years of study.

The Joy of Celibacy. This booklet examines how the unconscious is influenced by the sexual sell of modern advertising and suggests a five-minute celibacy break to help build awareness and self-knowledge.

Conversations with Swami Lakshmanjoo, Volume I: Aspects of Kashmir Shaivism. Edited transcripts of Alice Christensen's interviews with Swami Lakshmanjoo, talking about his childhood and early years in Yoga, plus some basic concepts in the philosophy of Kashmir Shaivism.

Conversations with Swami Lakshmanjoo, Volume II: Ethics of Yoga: The Yamas and Niyamas. Edited transcripts of Alice Christensen's dialogues with Swami Lakshmanjoo about these essential ethical guidelines in Yoga.

Audiotapes

Complete Relaxation and Meditation with Alice Christensen. A two-audiocassette program that features three guided meditation sessions of varying lengths, including instruction in a seated posture, plus a discussion of meditation experiences.

The "I Love You" Meditation Technique. This technique begins with the experience of a more conscious connection with the breath through love. It then extends this feeling throughout the body and mind in relaxation and meditation. This tape teaches you the beauty of loving yourself and it removes unseen fear.

Videotapes

Basic Yoga. A complete introduction to Yoga that includes exercise, breathing, and relaxation and meditation techniques. Provides detailed instruction in all the techniques including variations for more or less flexibility, plus a special limbering routine and back-strengthening exercises. Features a 30-minute practice session in a Yoga class setting for a convenient routine to do daily.

Conversations with Swami Lakshmanjoo. A set of three videotapes in which Alice Christensen introduces Swami Lakshmanjoo and talks with him about his background, the philosophy of Kashmir Shaivism, and other topics in Yoga. (Some material corresponds to Volume I of the book *Aspects of Kashmir Shaivism* described above in "Books.")

The Yamas and Niyamas: A Videotape Study Program. A complete set of 25 videotapes of Alice Christensen's comprehensive lectures on the ethical guidelines that form the cornerstone of Yoga philosophy and practice.

The Hero in Yoga: A Videotape Study Program. A series of 24 videotaped lectures by Alice Christensen on Joseph Campbell's landmark text *The Hero with a Thousand Faces*, showing how the adventure of the hero, represented in mythologies all over the globe, parallels the Yoga student's search for self-actualization.

INDEX

Boldface numbers indicate illustrations.

ABOUT THE AMERICAN YOGA ASSOCIATION

The American Yoga Association teaches a comprehensive and balanced program of Yoga that includes the Hatha Yoga exercises and breathing techniques as well as meditation. Rather than stressing physical culture for its own sake, our core curriculum acknowledges the deeper possibilities of Yoga by teaching meditation and by encouraging the inner-directed awareness that eventually leads to greater self-knowledge. This reliance on individual experience and feeling is a central theme in the science of Yoga, and it underlies the philosophical system of Kashmir Shaivism, which supports our line of teaching.

Our goal is to offer the highest quality Yoga instruction possible. There are two American Yoga Association Centers in the United States.

ABOUT THE AUTHOR

Alice Christensen stands out as a Yoga teacher with the rare ability to make the often-complex ideas and techniques of Yoga accessible to our Western outlook and lifestyle. She established the American Yoga Association in 1968, then the first and only nonprofit organization in the United States dedicated to education in Yoga.

She has consistently presented Yoga in a clear, classical manner for more than 40 years. She presents Yoga without dogma or prescription, as a potent avenue for individual inquiry. She has designed programs of Yoga that can be used to enhance any lifestyle. Whether to maintain health or to explore the nature of the self, her programs can be used to achieve a wide range of goals.